Profitable Dental Practice

8 strategies for building a practice that everyone loves to visit

SECOND EDITION

PHILIP NEWSOME

Honorary Clinical Associate Professor, Faculty of Dentistry,
University of Hong Kong
Specialist Prosthodontist

and

CHRIS BARROW

Writer, Speaker, Coach, Mentor
Founding Partner, 7connections

Foreword by
TREVOR W FERGUSON
Dean of The Faculty of General Dental Practitioners (UK)
The Royal College of Surgeons of England

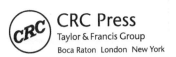

CRC Press
Taylor & Francis Group
Boca Raton London New York

CRC Press is an imprint of the
Taylor & Francis Group, an **informa** business

CRC Press
Taylor & Francis Group
6000 Broken Sound Parkway NW, Suite 300
Boca Raton, FL 33487-2742

No claim to original U.S. Government works

ISBN-13: 9781846197772 (pbk)

This book contains information obtained from authentic and highly regarded sources. While all reasonable efforts have been made to publish reliable data and information, neither the author[s] nor the publisher can accept any legal respon-sibility or liability for any errors or omissions that may be made. The publishers wish to make clear that any views or opinions expressed in this book by individual editors, authors or contributors are personal to them and do not neces-sarily reflect the views/opinions of the publishers. The information or guidance contained in this book is intended for use by medical, scientific or health-care professionals and is provided strictly as a supplement to the medical or other professional's own judgement, their knowledge of the patient's medical history, relevant manufacturer's instructions and the appropriate best practice guidelines. Because of the rapid advances in medical science, any information or advice on dosages, procedures or diagnoses should be independently verified. The reader is strongly urged to consult the relevant national drug formulary and the drug companies' and device or material manufacturers' printed instructions, and their websites, before administering or utilizing any of the drugs, devices or materials mentioned in this book. This book does not indicate whether a particular treatment is appropriate or suitable for a particular individual. Ultimately it is the sole responsibility of the medical professional to make his or her own professional judgements, so as to advise and treat patients appropriately. The authors and publishers have also attempted to trace the copyright holders of all mate-rial reproduced in this publication and apologize to copyright holders if permission to publish in this form has not been obtained. If any copyright material has not been acknowledged please write and let us know so we may rectify in any future reprint.

**Visit the Taylor & Francis Web site at
http://www.taylorandfrancis.com**

**and the CRC Press Web site at
http://www.crcpress.com**

British Library Cataloguing in Publication Data
A catalogue record for this book is available from the British Library.

Typeset by Darkriver Design, Auckland, New Zealand

Contents

Foreword to second edition

In 1986 yet another young and enthusiastic graduate left University with a BDS. There were few house jobs and for most of my generation, as had been the case before and since, gainful employment was to be found in general practice.

Looking back, qualifying as a dentist was the easy bit. As undergraduates we had received only tacit training in General Dental Practice and this was limited to running an 'intercalated clinic' rather than any aspect of business. Never was business or money discussed. Training was purely clinical. We were after all clinicians?

During the course of my career more and more emphasis has come to be placed on the 'business of dentistry'. Yet it cannot be said that training has evolved to complement this considerable skill required of practitioners. To add further pressure consumer organisations have become ever more vocal when criticising dentists for their financial activities and regulators have taken an ever more stringent position, often increasing practice costs with a level of compliance now required in the UK almost unsurpassed in any other profession.

It is often quoted that 95% plus of dentistry is delivered in the High Street. Clinicians who own a dental practice are small business owners. However, many are poorly trained for this critical aspect of their professional career. A number remain reluctant business people and some find it extremely difficult to blend clinical practice and ethical standards with business. They may sell their practice prematurely whilst others allow the practice to become an overbearing and occasionally debilitating influence on their professional and personal lives.

Against this backdrop it might seem that the situation is hopeless? My own experience (and of others) has been far from that. It is from my nearly 30 years as a dental businessman and clinician my belief has formed that dentists can run ethical profitable practices. So it is for this reason I am very pleased to be able to write the Foreword to this second edition of *Profitable Dental Practice*.

So how can it be done? Where is this Utopia to be found?

In the clinical arena the clinician must be confident and proficient in their clinical skills and patient management. Clinical teaching emphasises technically perfect dentistry, which is required at all times. However, indiscriminate use of technical skills may only lead to short-term outcomes with dentists trying to save teeth rather than manage long-term viable dentitions. In a consumer-driven society patients (or customers) expect value for money and that treatment delivered will have a reasonable lifetime. The successful clinician will realise this and manage patient expectations and only deliver treatment which they are competent to do. Additional clinical skills can be learnt over time but a reflective, honest and open approach to personal and professional development is essential. So-called 'soft' or communication skills are also necessary tools when discussing difficult and sometimes complicated treatment plans, especially when it is so important to gain valid consent. An empathy and understanding of patients' needs and wants with an ability to blend these with that which will deliver predictable clinical outcomes is vital.

Then of course dentists need to develop the business skills which they will require to run a successful profitable business. It is only through this they can hope to provide the basis from which they can deliver the high-quality clinical services which so many yearn to do. It is worth reflecting on that many disciplinary cases brought before regulators have their origins in the financial pressures clinicians have found themselves wrestling with in practice.

The business of dentistry requires skills not only in finance and law, but human resources, business planning and development, organisation, communication and leadership, marketing and IT, to name but a few. Interestingly, as with clinical skills the dentist may not possess all necessary business attributes in depth but needs to know when to delegate and refer these to others. Whether running a single or group of practices the ability to build a team, to lead and drive a business forward is essential. It cannot simply be assumed that every graduate possesses these skills or that they will acquire them ad hoc as their career progresses. With the rise of corporate dentistry it is my view that if the profession wishes to remain financially autonomous then more young practitioners will have to recognise the need for these skills much earlier in their careers than hitherto, and become as proficient in them as clinical dentistry.

So it is essential that clinical and business skills are not seen as mutually exclusive and that a profitable dental practice lies in a combination of both. This book also provides a combination. Phil Newsome, an undergraduate teacher and international speaker not only on clinical dentistry, but how that needs to integrate with the business of dentistry (almost uniquely for a university-based clinician) and Chris Barrow, who has over 20 years cajoled and encouraged many UK dental business owners to learn to not only sell themselves and their practice but to reflect and develop themselves personally.

Whilst no single book or educational event can provide 'The' solution I would however commend this book both to the young graduate aspiring to

Foreword to first edition

Some would say that the dental practitioner faces an unenviable challenge in having to be a healthcare professional at the same time as trying to run a business. There can be conflicts between the two from time to time, when the need of any business to create profits can get in the way of the ethical imperative for any healthcare professional to keep the best interests of the patient paramount at all times.

At first sight this seems to be an uneasy partnership, but it is one that is mirrored by the partnership between Phil Newsome and Chris Barrow – two unusual people with different professional careers that were themselves unusual in their own way. This book is the result of a fascinating synergy between an academically-based dentist who has always been fascinated by the world of business and marketing, and a former insurance salesman and independent financial adviser who has been fascinated by the untapped business opportunities in the professions generally, but dentistry in particular.

It is also a fusion between two people who have spent their lives in communication – one in teaching undergraduate dental students in the day job (and anyone else that would listen the rest of the time), and the other whose speciality has become coaching, and teaching people to bring out the best in themselves and others.

We should not be too surprised, therefore, to find ourselves enjoying the fruit of this fortunate union. The book is written unashamedly for dentists who have been too busy to listen to their inner voices, too busy providing dentistry to think about the benefits that patients might want from it, and too busy to step back from the day-to-day pressures of dental practice to recognise the rich vein of opportunity that has been coursing, unnoticed, through every day of their professional lives. The messages are powerfully and effectively conveyed. You won't agree with them all – at least, not today – but few of us are comfortable when our views are challenged. Professional people tend to be particularly sensitive, especially when their ethics, skills and standards of patient care are being questioned.

But, I would invite you to accept that the book stops you in your tracks only to facilitate the process of making tomorrow better than yesterday. The work of the dental profession is changing at a remarkable rate, and the skills we all learned at dental school – whenever that was – are no longer enough to provide the platform for a successful career in dental practice.

The irony is that technical, clinical skills are only a very small part of the toolkit that one needs in order to be successful in the real world of dental practice. This realisation comes quicker to some than to others. Yet the soft skills of communication and patient care in the broad, holistic sense, will make a much greater difference to our professional lives than the next piece of fancy dental equipment, or 'wonder material' or new technique. These shooting stars in the dental firmament fade surprisingly quickly, but the core skills outlined in this book will last a lifetime.

Despite its title – and I suppose even books need to sell themselves – the book is about a lot more than profit in the traditional sense. Paradoxically, a lot of this book is actually about loss – lost profits, yes, but also loss of balance in one's personal life, wasted time, lost staff, lost patients, lost potential patients, and lost opportunities in patients you have been treating for years. Above all else, one is forced to realise how much fun and personal satisfaction there is in finding that elusive formula that allows you to be a successful businessman or businesswoman who happens to be a dentist.

If it does nothing else other than persuade you that you are selling yourself (and your patients) short if you continue to squander the time you spend with those with whom you share your life – at home and at work – then I suspect the authors will reflect upon a job well done.

Kevin Lewis
Dental Director
Dental Protection Ltd
Medical Protection Society
June 2004

Preface to second edition

What is success? One thing that may be said with some certainty is that it can and does mean different things to different people. Financial gain probably springs to mind first, but your career isn't entirely about money is it? For most people it is something deeper, something central to your core, having your say, making things happen, personal fulfilment, the recognition of others . . . all of these and more contribute to the much-desired but often elusive condition that we call success. While there may be many ways to achieve success it does seem that those organisations that are considered to be successful do share a number of common characteristics. This book looks at how those characteristics apply to the profession of dentistry, at what it takes to create and sustain a successful dental practice. There exist literally hundreds of dental practices, and while most of them provide their owners with a reasonable living, only a small number could be described as being truly successful, flourishing organisations. The eight strategies described in this book mesh together to provide a blueprint for anyone wishing to develop a thriving dental practice, one that enhances the lives of everyone involved with it – patients, support staff and of course the dentist. A brief explanation of each chapter follows.

Introduction: The changing face of dental practice

This chapter looks at how dental practice has changed in recent times and, indeed, since the first edition of this book was published in 2004. It examines what impact factors such as improved treatment modalities, deregulation, the rise of corporate dentistry, direct access and the growth in consumerism have had upon the profession. The case will be made that in such a rapidly changing business environment the strong will get stronger and the weak will struggle to survive.

Strategy 1: Construct a powerful three-year vision

Dreams don't usually come true by accident. Success in any walk of life is more likely to happen if you can envisage that success and then plan for it to happen. Key features of this planning process include a clearly articulated personal and professional mission statement coupled with specific goals covering every aspect of one's life – financial, business, family, social, physical, intellectual and spiritual.

Strategy 2: Plan the time to plan

One of the biggest obstacles in the process of making transformational change is a perceived 'lack of time'. There is no such thing as 'lack of time' – there is only an inability to prioritise time effectively. Failing to plan is planning to fail – allocating time, well in advance, for strategic thinking, strategic planning and strategic action is one of the most important habits of the successful dental team leader.

Strategy 3: Control your finances

No practice, whatever its size or nature, can be considered to be truly successful without a firm commitment to maintaining its financial health. This means living within your means, preparing budgets for both business and personal expenditure a year in advance, preparing management accounts at the end of each month, comparing actual versus budget accounts and taking corrective action on a monthly basis. Pricing strategy should be carefully calculated to cover the fixed costs and overheads of running the business, to provide the owner's desired income and to allow for the setting aside of monies for the future.

Strategy 4: Lead a championship support team

Successful dental practices show clear evidence of effective leadership and the creation of a practice culture that is compatible with the practice owner's core vision. Our belief is that you should spend 80% of your time focusing on your unique ability of building relationships with the right type of patients, to help them identify and solve their current and future problems and aspirations. The remaining 20% of your time should be spent leading the support staff who then have responsibility for carrying out everything else – namely, financial control, sales strategy, marketing and day-to-day operational control. Without exception, all successful dental practices possess a keen, motivated, highly trained, well-rewarded, empowered and harmonious team.

Strategy 5: Deliver world-class customer service

The traditional 'doctor knows best' approach to dental practice has no place nowadays – patients expect to be involved in any decisions that affect them. Successful practices recognise this and therefore do all they can to understand more about their patients, their likes, dislikes and motivation, and in so doing maximise the practice's ability to attract and retain the best patients. Patients are no longer going to tolerate the conditions that exist in many practices.

Poor location, difficult access, substandard décor, low staff morale, out-of-date equipment and lousy literature will simply drive patients into the arms of those who are willing to invest in success.

Strategy 6: Refine your selling skills

Like it or not, a practice is a sales operation and everybody who works in it works in sales. Not hard, pushy, aggressive sales but soft, ethical sales – creating an environment in which patients want to buy. The majority of dentists have very little idea about the psychology of selling and are pretty good at keeping their products and services a secret from the people who could buy them. A sales organisation should have clearly visible targets that should be communicated to the support team on a regular basis. Part of the team's remuneration should be linked to performance against these targets so that the whole team becomes empowered by the process of achieving targets, while at the same time maintaining professional standards.

Strategy 7: Create a low-cost marketing engine

Many dentists say that they have tried a marketing technique at some stage, but stopped 'because it didn't work'. Rarely though is there a marketing plan – a systematic low-cost approach where events are scheduled up to a year in advance and delegated to the support team. Successful practices understand the need for a comprehensive and ongoing marketing strategy involving not only obvious promotional strategies but also an understanding that marketing is built around *all* the day-to-day interactions or 'moments of truth' that take place between the practice and its patients.

Strategy 8: Maintain a balance between work, rest and play

It doesn't matter how much profit you are generating from your practice if your life is dysfunctional, if you are always stressed, if you are frequently in a state of chronic fatigue, if your family and friends don't know who you are, if you never seem to have enough time for yourself.

Philip Newsome
Chris Barrow
January 2014

About the authors

Philip Newsome graduated with honours from Leeds Dental School in 1976. After a number of years in general dental practice he returned to academic life at Leeds before moving to the University of Hong Kong's Faculty of Dentistry in 1986. His time is now divided between private practice, writing and speaking engagements. He holds an FDS and MRD from the Royal College of Surgeons of Edinburgh and is on the UK and Hong Kong specialist lists for prosthodontics. He also has an MBA from the University of Warwick Business School and a PhD from the University of Bradford Management Centre. In 2013 he was awarded an honorary Fellowship of the Faculty of General Dental Practitioners (UK) for his contribution to the profession.

Chris Barrow has been active as a consultant, trainer and coach to the UK dental profession for over 20 years. Naturally direct, assertive and determined, he has the ability to reach conclusions quickly, as well as the sharp reflexes and lightness of touch to innovate, change tack and push boundaries. As a speaker he is dynamic, energetic and charismatic. Chris spent the first 17 years of his working life in the corporate sector and followed this with 26 years of self-employment. The different dynamics of both worlds have given him the valuable gift of knowing how to operate – and communicate – in both. In 1987 Chris was active in the establishment of the Institute for Financial Planning, an organisation representing the first fee-based financial planners; Chris specialised in working with small businesses. In 1993 Chris decided to make the transition to business coaching and became one of the first UK students at Coach University, from where he graduated as a certified coach. Recognising the opportunity in the dental profession, 1997 saw the creation of The Dental Business School and the development of a 12-month business coaching programme for dental practice owners and their teams, delivered to over 400 UK dental practices in the following 10 years. In October 2008, Chris became Director of Private Sector Development at Integrated Dental Holdings Ltd and now acts as an occasional Non-Executive Director for dental corporates as well as continuing his freelance consultancy work for corporates, primary care trusts and independent practices. His main focus now is on 7connections, a privately owned company that specialises in training, consultancy, coaching and mentorship in independent dentistry and also takes minority equity positions in private practices.

Acknowledgements

My contribution to this book is based on all the things I have learnt and on all the mistakes I have made over the many years since I entered dental school. I have been so fortunate to have worked with some of the wisest, most knowledgeable and downright funny people you could ever wish to meet. My first years in dental practice with Peter Hamlyn were wonderful times, as was the period I spent with John Dyson. Those years in practice taught me that as dentists we care for people first, mouths second. During my academic career, Professor Richard Walker stands out as a mentor, friend and critic who taught me that you can do almost anything – as long as you do it with a smile, charm and wit. Equally, Professor Ted Renson and Professor Fred Smales have been tremendously supportive, as has Professor Gillian Wright.

Philip Newsome

In his book *True Success*, philosopher Tom Morris defined success as 'doing what you want to do, when you want to do it and with the people you want to do it with.' Not exactly Shakespeare but it makes the point. In considering my own definition of success, I would replace the word 'want' with the word 'love' – because I truly love the work I do, the times when I do work and the people I work with. Which allows me to acknowledge all the fantastic clients I have worked with over the years and who have been my priceless R & D team, telling me when my ideas were awesome, OK or just crazy and impossible. Then there are the giants whose shoulders I have stood on – the authors of the many books and speakers at conferences who have inspired and enlightened. The friends, both professional and personal, who have cared enough to listen. The team who have supported me from backstage over the years, tolerating and compensating for my weaknesses. The family who have always been there and always will be. I dedicate my contribution to this work to those I love.

Chris Barrow

CHAPTER ONE

Introduction: The changing face of dental practice

Whoever desires constant success must change his conduct with the times.

Niccolò Machiavelli

The latter part of the twentieth century saw far-reaching changes in the economies of most westernised countries. Such modern economies are based more and more on the production and consumption of increasingly differentiated goods and services. Few sectors have escaped this shift in emphasis and that includes the practice of dentistry. For many years the vast majority of dental procedures performed in the UK were done so under the National Health Service (NHS) umbrella, with treatment costs heavily subsidised by the government. There wasn't too much choice in the kind of treatments being offered to patients, and even less choice in the way that this treatment was provided. Most patients received their dental care in converted residential properties and the treatment itself, if we are honest with ourselves, usually centred on a mixture of amalgams in posterior teeth, composites (or more likely silicate cements) in anteriors, extractions, a quick scale and polish (with little thought to any long-term management of the patient's periodontal condition), metal-based full crowns, partial dentures, perhaps conventional bridgework and at the end of the road . . . traditional full dentures. The relationship between dentist and patient was paternalistic at best, with patients usually having little say in what treatment was provided – 'they aren't really paying for it so why should they have a say?' was an attitude prevalent at the time. Going 'private' was an option taken up by a very small percentage of the public and usually only by those people living in the most affluent regions of the country.

While some cynics might argue that in many practices up and down the country this scenario has hardly altered, there is no doubt that times are changing. Treatment options have increased dramatically and the approach to care is now aimed more towards prevention than mere repair and is increasingly patient-driven rather than entirely dentist-directed, with a greater emphasis on elective dentistry in the form of whitening, tooth-coloured fillings, laminate veneers, implants, and so on. Since the events of the 1980s and early 1990s many dentists have opted out of the NHS and are now providing dental care that is financed independently. New corporate players, with a more retail-oriented outlook, have sensed an opportunity and have entered the market with considerable financial backing from a variety of financial backers. This introductory chapter looks at these various trends and explores how they have shaped, and continue to shape, the profession. The concurrence of these trends has created an environment in which an ever-increasing number of 'savvy' dentists are able to run extremely successful practices while at the same time providing the sort of care and work environment that could only have been dreamt of even a short while back.

THE CHANGING ROLE OF THE DENTIST

Fundamental advances in oral healthcare have resulted in a far greater emphasis on scientific, evidence-based treatments. Take, for example, the recently adopted National Institute for Health and Care Excellence guidelines on the use of antibiotic cover in dentistry. These turned conventional wisdom on its head and have seen the almost total elimination of the once ubiquitous prophylactic antibiotic cover in UK dental practice.[1] Research has done much to clarify the biological and behavioural mechanisms involved in oral health and the prevention of disease – primarily dental caries and periodontal disease. Successive Adult Dental Health Surveys have shown that the oral health of UK adults has improved significantly over recent decades. For example, the proportion of adults in England with visible coronal caries has fallen from 46% in 1998 to 28% in 2009 while the proportion of edentulous adults in England has fallen from 28% in 1978 to 6% in 2009.[2] Nowadays, people are rendered edentulous at a rate that is almost too small to measure. Many millions have been converted from recurring emergency extractions to regular check-ups. In short, a massive number of people now enjoy the benefits of good dental health.

With this reduction in gross disease, in a more dentally aware population, a larger proportion of a dentist's work is now elective in nature, dealing with matters of poor appearance and impaired function rather than the simple alleviation of pain. Greater emphasis is also being placed upon evidence-based dentistry. In tandem with these changes, technological developments in areas such as dental materials, pharmacology and treatment modalities have resulted in a much wider range of treatment options. Most of these procedures are much more technique-sensitive than their predecessors – for example, consider placing an implant compared with providing a partial denture, or inserting a posterior composite as opposed to an amalgam. Because of this added complexity these techniques demand a coordinated team approach if they are to be successful – 'team' meaning not only the dentist and his or her chair-side assistant but also hygienists and technical support, even front-desk staff have an important role to play by helping us to communicate better with patients as well understanding and even modifying their expectations.

All of these changes have a number of important implications for the way we work. While ever higher standards of clinical practice are required of the dentist and other members of the dental team, clinical practice will increasingly centre on prevention, control and self-care strategies based on knowledge of general health and the lifestyle of individual patients – for example, counselling patients to wear mouthguards while playing sports. Such preventive-oriented approaches towards care usually require a fundamental shift in the patient's behaviour and the modern dentist (together with his or her staff) is therefore called upon to be more aware of, and more sensitive to, issues concerning patient compliance and motivation.

Keeping 'up to date' with all these changes makes dental education a vital and continuing process, demanding more commitment from the dental practitioner than in the past, when the pace of change was much slower and when many a dentist would seemingly pass from graduation to retirement virtually without ever learning anything new. In 2002, in recognition of this need for dentists to stay up to date, the General Dental Council (GDC) implemented its programme of compulsory continuing professional development (CPD), with CPD defined as:

> *study, training, courses, seminars, reading and other activities undertaken by a dentist, which could reasonably be expected to advance his or her professional development as a dentist.*[3]

The advent of compulsory core subjects in 2007 further strengthened this approach. Successful dentists know all too well that keeping *meaningfully* up to date is a must, not something to which they pay mere lip-service and they will therefore devote time, energy and resources to do so. They will also encourage, even insist, all their staff do the same and indeed in 2008 the GDC made CPD compulsory for all dental care professionals.

Given the rapid changes in the way dental care is being delivered, CPD should also embrace not only 'hard' treatment modalities, but also 'softer' interpersonal and behavioural aspects of dental care as well as a knowledge of business management methods which helps to blend all these disparate parts together to produce a successful dental practice. In 2008 the GDC issued *Guidance on Principles of Management Responsibility* offering direction for those dental professionals with management responsibility.[4] It is widely accepted that most graduating dentists sadly do not possess the requisite knowledge and skills to become competent practice principals and little seems to have changed in this regard since the publication in 1999 of one British Dental Association (BDA) survey looking into the views of over 1000 young dentists (that is those qualifying after 1987) who, while feeling well-prepared for general practice in most clinical aspects, considered themselves ill-prepared in areas such as staff management, business and finance.[5] The dentist's role is clearly changing and the modern professional has so much more to contend with than counterparts, say, 20 or 30 years earlier. This was clearly articulated in a letter published in the *British Dental Journal* in the spring of 2013, in which the author, a retiring dentist, rather cynically observed:

> *Forty years ago my job description was dental surgeon; today my job title is performer and provider of primary dental care for the local PCT [primary care trust], lead in child protection, lead for cross-infection control, radiological protection supervisor, health and safety supervisor, fire warden, lead for information governance, lead for staff training, and environmental cleaning operative.*[6]

Perhaps fortunate then for the writer of that letter that he is retiring, as there lurks on the horizon a further sea change in the shape of *revalidation*. The publication in 2007 of the government's White Paper *Trust, Assurance and Safety*[7] proposed that all health regulators are required to develop a system of revalidation. Accordingly, the GDC has been working for some time towards a system in which a dentist is obligated to prove that he or she is fit to stay on the *Dentists Register*.[8] Compulsory CPD can now be seen as a first step of a far wider process in which the onus is on the dentist to demonstrate not only that he or she has undertaken some postgraduate courses but also that he or she complies with the standards set by the GDC throughout his or her professional life. It is proposed that revalidation will encompass four domains: (1) clinical, (2) professionalism, (3) management or leadership and (4) communication. At the time of writing it is not clear how dentists in different sectors, such as academia, will be assessed. Not surprisingly, a number in the profession view this whole exercise as yet another set of disproportionate, onerous, bureaucratic impositions, as one frustrated contributor to an online discussion group noted:[9]

> *Another idea that sounds good on paper, but in reality is not necessary. Surely revalidation shouldn't apply to anyone with a clear record with no complaints? What big problem do we have in dentistry that revalidation will fix. Revalidation is very likely to degenerate into yet another box ticking exercise, instantly increasing expenses to patients and dentistry providers, and reducing access to dental care. We're already being revalidated and regulated and nickel and dimed to death.*

The difficulty is that revalidation will happen. Forward-thinking dentists will not wait to be told to keep up to date and abreast of all relevant developments in their profession. Unfortunately, such developments and shifts in philosophy are often slow to be adopted by the majority of dentists, but those who have embraced this new paradigm of care are reaping the rewards in terms of increased satisfaction – not only their own but also that of their staff and, crucially, their patients. A number of dentists have seized upon the opportunities presented by entering specific niches within the profession – for example, in areas such as orthodontics and implants. This, unsurprisingly, has created a backlash from specialists in these fields who feel undermined and fear a lowering of clinical standards.

Patient satisfaction is, as we will see, one of the ultimate goals for any successful practice. For it to happen, the practice principal must see himself as more than just a dentist, he must also be a visionary. Dreams don't usually come true by accident. Success in any walk of life is more likely to happen if you can envisage that success and then plan for it to happen. Key features of this planning process include a clearly articulated personal and professional mission statement coupled with specific goals covering every aspect of one's life – financial, business, family, social, physical, intellectual and spiritual.

GREATER EMPHASIS ON A TEAM APPROACH TO PROVISION OF DENTAL CARE

Successful dental practices show clear evidence of effective leadership and the creation of a working culture that is compatible with the practice owner's core vision. Almost without exception, all successful dental practices possess a keen, motivated, highly-trained, well-rewarded, empowered and harmonious staff, which has traditionally comprised receptionists, back-room staff, dental nurses, hygienists and, of course, dentists, but which increasingly includes practice managers and treatment coordinators, among others. It is a key management task to see that such a team is established.

The need for a team approach to dentistry received considerable attention throughout the 1990s, primarily in the various reports published by the likes of the Nuffield Foundation[10] and the GDC.[11] Generally speaking, there has been a move away from small, often single-handed, practices with minimal support staff, in favour of larger group practices with a corresponding emphasis on the 'team' approach to care. In addition to the advantages a larger team can bring in terms of the range and flexibility of services that can be offered to patients, expanded practices are better placed to take advantage of economies of scale, as both fixed and non-fixed costs can be spread over more dentists and surgeries. From the description we have given here thus far, it may seem that this trend is entirely one-way, an assumption that would, however, be misleading. A number of dentists have 'downsized' from larger practices (with one or more associates) back to single-handed practices, albeit with a strong emphasis on quality of care provided by a small team of dedicated staff. It appears that for some dentists the task of finding associates who share the same vision of dental practice proves to be just too difficult in a climate characterised by a shortage of dentists, or more pertinently a shortage of dentists they would want to have working in their practice. One dentist expressed this view thus:*

> *The second best day in your working life is when you take on an associate . . . the best day is when they leave.*

Ten years ago, when the first edition of this book was published, we discussed the perceived and actual shortage of dentists in the UK. This is less of an issue now and as a result there is a significant and continued reduction in associate remuneration. This is partly a result of there being more dentists in the marketplace and partly because, from a business standpoint, practice owners simply cannot justify the high percentages previously being paid.

While the rate of change towards a more integrated team approach is first and foremost a commercial response to the need for higher levels of care and service being demanded by the public, it is also widely appreciated in the profession that there is a need to clarify and enhance the roles played by all types of dental ancillary staff. The Dental Auxiliaries Review Group, which was set up by the GDC to explore the future role of ancillary dental staff, published its report in May 1998 and concluded that 'dental care in the next century will be provided by a multi-skilled team comprising members of the dental profession

---

* Anonymous. Personal communication.

and professions complementary to dentistry, all led by a dentist'.[12] It was anticipated there would be new classes of operating auxiliaries who would carry out
the more routine aspects of dentistry as part of teams directed by a dentist,
probably one per team, whose role it would be to do the treatment planning
and the more sophisticated aspects of dentistry. This gained further momen-
tum in 2008 when the GDC introduced mandatory registration for all dental
care professionals, dental nurses, dental technicians, clinical dental technicians,
hygienists, therapists and orthodontic therapists. At the time of writing, over
63 000 dental care professionals are registered with the GDC. There is, however,
one potential fly in the proverbial ointment with the announcement by the
GDC in March of 2013 that it would remove its barrier to direct access for some
dental care professionals. In the past, every member of the dental team had to
work on the prescription of a dentist. This meant that patients had to be seen
by a dentist before being treated by any other member of the dental team. This
latest move represents a complete *volte-face* by the GDC and clearly contradicts
earlier GDC initiatives (as discussed earlier). It appears to have arisen through
pressure from the Office of Fair Trading and is being vehemently opposed by
the BDA, whose view was very clearly stated in a statement released on the date
the decision was announced:

> *This is a misguided decision that fails to consider best practice in essential continuity of*
> *care, patient choice and cost-effectiveness, and weakens teamworking in dentistry which*
> *is demonstrated to be in patients' best interests. Dental hygienists and therapists are*
> *highly-valued and competent members of the dental team, but they do not undertake*
> *the full training that dentists do and on their own are not able to provide the holistic,*
> *comprehensive care that patients need and expect. Our fear is that this could lead to*
> *health problems being missed in patients who choose to access hygiene and therapy*
> *appointments directly.*[13]

It remains to be seen exactly what effect this move will have on the dental
marketplace, but at first sight it does appear to undo all the effort put into
promoting the concept of the dentist-led team, which focuses on the need for
patients to see a dentist first for a comprehensive oral health assessment and
treatment plan.

CONSUMER DEMAND

Thinking of patients as consumers is something of a double-edged sword. On
the one hand, dentistry, along with all the other healthcare services, is finding its clientele to be more demanding in terms of the expected range and

quality of services, as well as the availability of information about those services. Increasingly, people want more say about their health and health services and are demanding the best care for themselves and their families, together with greater choice in that care. The profession should not see this as being a negative development. On the contrary, it is a plus for the profession to have patients who don't look on themselves as passive recipients of care and who instead demand a greater involvement in the process of care. The fact too that patients are paying a much larger percentage of the total treatment cost than in the past has clearly had an effect, in that they expect to know much more about what exactly they are receiving for their money. Patients are also more likely to express their dissatisfaction whenever they are unhappy with any aspect of the service provided and this has led to a far more litigious environment than at any time in the past. Indeed, one of the most noticeable trends over the past two decades has been a dramatic increase in the number of patient complaints against dentists. It is debatable whether this is because of a moral decline in the profession, or because modern dentistry is so much more complicated nowadays that more things can go wrong or possibly because the public are more inclined to complain in these modern times. The truth is likely to contain elements of all three of these. What is undeniable is that in recent years there has been a staggering growth in the number of disciplinary cases being heard by the GDC. In response, in 2005, the GDC published *Standards for Practice*[14] effectively a road-map detailing the responsibilities of a dental profession. This was updated in 2013 and appeared as the subtly re-named *Standards for the Dental Team*[15] featuring the following nine key principles.

1. Put patients' interests first.
2. Communicate effectively with patients.
3. Obtain valid consent.
4. Maintain and protect patients' information.
5. Have a clear and effective complaints procedure.
6. Work with colleagues in a way that serves the interests of patients.
7. Maintain, develop and work within your professional knowledge and skills.
8. Raise concerns if patients are at risk.
9. Make sure your personal behaviour maintains patients' confidence in you and the dental profession.

The emphasis in this document on 'softer skills' and a patient orientation is clear, and on its launch GDC Chief Executive Evlynne Gilvarry observed:

> Patients have told us clearly what they expect when they seek dental treatment. The new standards reflect those expectations and guide the dental profession in meeting them.

The GDC clearly hope that this initiative will go some way to quelling the rising number of disciplinary cases being heard. The figures speak for themselves. For example, in 1987 the total number of hearing days scheduled by the GDC amounted to around 20. By 2012 this had mushroomed to more than 1019.[16]

Proactive companies in other industries do not see such consumerism as a threat but, rather, an opportunity to improve on their offer to consumers. As one Dell computer advertisement put it:[17]

> *To all our nit-picky, over-demanding, ask-awkward-questions customers. Thank you and keep up the good work.*

PUBLIC TRUST AND CONFIDENCE

Dentists need to embrace this new order and should not be defensive or feel threatened by it, even in the face of negative media coverage – especially when it comes to dentists who are seen to be abusing patient trust. Trust and confidence is a huge issue for most patients. Back in 1998 the *Reader's Digest* ran a story titled:

> *Can you trust your dentist? After all, the more treatment he recommends, the more money he makes. Our special investigation exposes some alarming practices.*[18]

Such media coverage upsets many in the profession and yet it is symptomatic of the fact that patients recognise all too well that they don't really understand what is 'good practice' in terms of much of the treatment provided. A variety of scandals down the years only reinforces the public view that some members of the profession are highly dubious charlatans and fraudsters, interested only in money. Successful practices are those that address the fundamental issue of trust by placing great emphasis on genuinely caring for patients in the widest sense of the word, by treating patients with respect, by going to the greatest lengths to communicate with them, and so on.

The other side of the 'consumer' coin is that the growing number of treatment options has led to an increase in demand for dental care. Paradoxically, much of this has been driven by the popular media, which has helped raise public awareness by emphasising the benefits of good oral health. Indeed, three out of four people in the UK now believe the health of their teeth and gums has a significant impact on their quality of life, according to the results of one survey.[19] The majority of people questioned (around two-thirds) felt that oral health had a major bearing on their appearance, comfort and how they ate, while just under half said they believed it was an important factor in terms of their self-confidence, social life and romantic relationships. The survey results confirmed that the mouth and teeth have a strong influence on the way people feel about themselves.

This growth in awareness of the positive aspects of good dental health has also been aided by the growth of private dentistry, which has provided patients with a wider range of choice, and dentists with more time to explain to the patient the pros and cons of these various treatment options. Patients nowadays have higher expectations, such as the possibility of avoiding extractions, and keeping teeth for life. They expect to be seen promptly and for treatment interventions to be successful. Overall they expect, and are demanding, a better quality of service.

Successful practices avoid the elitist and patronising approach characterised by 'doctor always knows best' – a style of dental practice that really has no place nowadays. Great practices emphasise how modern dentistry can benefit the individual and so involve the patient in any decision that might affect the patient's health, appearance, comfort and finances. Such practices do all they can to understand more about their patients, their likes, dislikes and motivation and in so doing maximise their own ability to attract and retain patients.

CLINICAL GOVERNANCE

While patients may not fully understand the technical aspects of the care they receive, they nevertheless do expect dentists to provide quality dental care, and rightly so. Clinical governance can be defined as a systematic method for ensuring that the patient's needs for quality of care are met. Proving you are as good as you think you are is not about demonstrating that you or your practice is perfect but that you organise and run your practice in a manner that encourages the pursuit of excellence in terms of meeting your patients' needs as well as their reasonable expectations. Successful practices appreciate the crucial importance of a practice-wide devotion to quality, not only in technical and clinical matters (e.g. formalising treatment plans and gaining effective consent) but also in the softer, non-technical aspects of care (such as effective communication). Increasingly, they also appreciate that the use of an independently verified system helps to identify areas in need of improvement and encourages the pursuit of excellence. Independent verification also goes a long way to reassuring patients who may have lost confidence in the profession.

All the major bodies connected to the practice of dentistry in the UK, from the GDC through to the major defence unions, agree that while such governance and related risk assessment is desirable, it is debatable how many practices would participate in such activities unless forced to do so by law. With all these concerns providing the backdrop, an independent regulator of health and adult social care services in England, the Care Quality Commission (CQC), was established in April 2009, and from April 2011 all primary dental services have had to register with the Commission. Registration is a legal licence to operate and, put simply, if dental practices are not registered then they will not be able to provide services. In order to become registered the provider must be deemed to be 'compliant' – that is, the provider must show that the service offered does indeed meet essential standards of safety and quality. The seemingly logical rationale behind the CQC is that when a practice has been assessed as compliant, then patients can expect the following:

- to be respected, involved and told what's happening at every stage
- care, treatment and support that meets your needs
- to be safe
- to be cared for by staff with the right skills to do their jobs properly
- your dental practice to routinely check the quality of its services.

However, the introduction of the CQC has been far from smooth and certainly has not been welcomed with any great enthusiasm by the profession, many of whose members view it as yet another unnecessary, centrally-imposed, ill-conceived, burden. *Dentistry* magazine reported that 'The introduction of compulsory registration with the CQC . . . triggered howls of protest from many dentists', and going on to report that 'The organisation was accused of inflicting chaos during a "farcical registration process" – with the threat of suspension for any dentists that failed to comply.'[20] Critics, including two parliamentary committees, have slammed the health watchdog as poorly led – and have questioned the decision to put dentists on the same footing as care homes. These views were mirrored by the BDA in a recent press release in which John Milne, Chair of the BDA's General Dental Practice Committee, observed:

> *The BDA has campaigned throughout this process for the myriad flaws inherent in the system to be addressed and for Government to apologise to dentists for the stress and difficulties that have been suffered. It's time for that long-overdue apology to be made. The magnitude of the problems . . . and the effect they have had on dentists should not be underestimated. Dentists have told us that the experience of CQC registration has led many of them to seriously consider their futures in dentistry. That is a sad reflection on an ill-conceived and woefully-flawed process.*[21]

Clearly this story has not yet reached its conclusion and only time will tell how it will end.

CHANGING APPROACHES TO DELIVERING DENTAL CARE

The most apparent change in the way dental care is delivered in the UK has been the move towards private dentistry, which had its roots in the dental profession's widespread dissatisfaction with the NHS fee structure of the early 1990s and in the changes introduced by the government at that time – ironically in an attempt to increase the number of patients seeking NHS dental care. The NHS was introduced in 1948 at a time when the oral health of the UK population was extremely poor. Many people had no teeth, dental decay was almost universal and infection was widespread. The basics of the system remained relatively unchanged well into the late 1980s, with dentists being rewarded according to how much they 'drilled and filled', not how well they did it or how appropriately they made their treatment decisions. There was growing concern that financial incentives were leading to over-treatment and following a review of these risks[22] a new contract was introduced in 1990 with an element of capitation (around 20%) that aimed at encouraging the registration of patients into continuing care. Initially the new arrangement was very successful in encouraging patients to register, perhaps too successful as it turned out. The amount of work carried out on these new patients was far greater than anticipated by the government, who sought to recoup the extra expenditure by imposing a drastic 7% cut in the fees payable to dentists. This was a pivotal moment for the UK dental profession. Given the changes already described – namely, the growing complexity and cost of treatment options, the need to employ more staff in order to create the all-important dental team, and, finally, a more demanding and knowledgeable public – many dentists decided the time had come to turn their back on the NHS if they were to maintain, and in most cases dramatically improve, the quality of care and range of services offered to patients. The work of Professor Cary Cooper around this time showed the degree of discontent felt by many dentists who agreed strongly with statements such as:

> The piecework system of remuneration should be refined so that dentists are not only paid for operative work but also for preventive work.
>
> Since dentists have to see as many patients as possible to earn a decent living, the quality of their work can suffer.[23]

Quoting a study conducted in the mid 1990s at the University of Manchester, Teresa Waddington[24] reported that the chief concern for dental practitioners was the uncertainty felt about possible further changes to the dental 'system', a concern voiced by virtually every dentist in the study.

> *The future of dentistry is so uncertain at the moment, you don't know where you're*
> *going to be in a couple of years' time.*
>
> *I suppose with most things it's the fear of the unknown. We're not really quite in*
> *control of what's going to happen next.* [24]

By the mid 1990s and with more dentists reducing their commitment to the NHS, access (or, more correctly, lack of access) to NHS dentists was becoming an increasingly important political issue. Against this backdrop of restlessness within the profession, a number of review bodies were established in an attempt to find solutions to the various problems plaguing general dental practice.[10,25,26] One of these, *NHS Dentistry: Options for Change*,[27] set out a vision for NHS dentistry with prevention at its heart and was widely supported by the profession. A variety of pilot schemes were tested, and in 2005 a new contract was launched that was based on a methodology for measuring dentists' activity and which, critically, had not previously been piloted.[28] The 2006 reforms featured three key issues.

1. Responsibility for planning and securing NHS dental services was now devolved to local primary care trusts.
2. The system of patient charges was changed, resulting in a reduction in the possible number of charges from around 400 to just three.
3. The mechanism by which dentists were to be paid to deliver NHS services was changed from one based on fees per items of service to one where providers would be paid an annual sum in return for delivering an agreed number of 'courses of treatment' or 'Units of Dental Activity' weighted by complexity.

A number of dentists were uncomfortable with the new arrangements and elected to convert to private practice. While the lost capacity was relatively small (4%), it served to exacerbate the already problematic access issues that had been growing since the early 1990s. It soon became clear that, rather than improving the situation, the new contract was making things worse. A *Daily Telegraph* headline from March 2007 said it all: 'Thousands Left Without Access to NHS Dentists'. The article noted:

> *The contract was intended to move dentists away from the 'drill and fill' image and*
> *give them more time for preventative work and taking on more NHS patients. But mis-*
> *calculations on the amount of money that fee-paying patients would bring meant that*
> *primary care trusts have told dentists to slow down because there was not enough money*
> *to pay for taking on new NHS patients.* [29]

The article also cited a BDA poll of 394 dentists, conducted one year after the new contracts started, showing clear dissatisfaction with the system. Eighty-five per cent of dentists surveyed did not think that the new contracts had improved patient access, and 95% did not think that the new contracts allowed them to spend more time with patients.

Clearly, many problems still existed and these lead to a further investigation into NHS dentistry conducted by the House of Commons Health Select Committee in 2008,[30] which in turn led to an extensive independent review, *NHS Dental Services in England*, led by Professor Jimmy Steele.[31] Subsequently, the government announced in 2010 that it would pilot three different models to help develop yet another NHS dental contract. This led to the development of a new body, the NHS Commissioning Board (NHSCB), which from April 2013 took over commissioning responsibility from primary care trusts for all NHS dental services – primary, community and secondary, including dental out-of-hours and urgent care. This will include commissioning dental services provided in high-street dental practices, community dental services, and dental services at general hospitals and dental hospitals. The stated aim of the NHSCB is to commission NHS dental services based on the local oral health needs assessment, which will be developed by public health teams in local authorities and will help determine the needs of local populations. It is hoped that the benefit of the NHSCB becoming a single commissioner for all dental services will be the ability to plan for and deliver more consistent standards, higher-quality services and better health outcomes for patients across the whole of England. A more consistent approach to commissioning and contract management will be implemented in order to deliver these improvements.

Over two decades on from the events that precipitated all these changes, the dental landscape has clearly changed dramatically in the UK, and yet, according to a comprehensive study carried out by the Office of Fair Trading in 2012, the majority of dental patients still receive NHS dental treatment.[32] Another study of the UK dental market noted that in 2011 there were approximately 29 500 dentists practising in primary care settings, with the vast majority offering NHS dental treatment or a combination of NHS and private dental treatment. Less than 10% of dentists (2500) were thought to carry out private treatment only.[33] The Office of Fair Trading study found that 66% of patients in England and Wales who had a regular dentist and had been to the dentist in the last two years reported that they received NHS dental treatment on their last visit. Twenty-three per cent reported that they had received private treatment and 10% reported that they received a mix of private and NHS dental treatment. More patients in Scotland reported receiving NHS dental treatment (75%), while fewer reported doing so in Northern Ireland (54%). Overall, the dentistry market in the UK has seen significant growth over recent years, its value rising by around 90% between the periods of 1999–2000 and 2009–10 and currently standing at an estimated £5.73 billion a year, with spending on NHS dental treatment accounting for approximately 58% of the market value and spending on private dental treatment accounting for the remaining 42%.[33]

Compare these figures with 1996–97 when NHS fees stood at £1.6 billion (71%) and private fees at £0.6 billion (29%) and it can be seen that the size of the whole market has grown massively. However, while the cash value of the NHS has almost exactly doubled in that time, the private sector has quad-rupled during the same period. These results clearly show that NHS dentistry is still alive and kicking, despite reports of its imminent demise, but equally there seems to be little doubt that the trend towards higher-priced and, one hopes, higher-quality care will also continue. That said, the recent economic downturn has undoubtedly had an impact on dentistry. While growth in the market was running at around 4% per annum from 2000 onwards, it slowed to 1% in 2008–09 and 2% in 2009–10.[33]

The move away from NHS-funded dental care has seen many dentists find-ing it convenient for both themselves and their patients to make use of the funding framework offered by one of a number of third-party schemes, with capitation plans by far the largest source of such funding for dentistry in the UK. Such capitation plans are based on a contract between the patient and the dentist to provide continuing routine care in exchange for a regular monthly payment or premium. Denplan, the largest of these schemes, offers a private capitation plan with, at the time of writing, approximately 1.8 million subscrib-ers and over 6500 UK dentists enrolled in the Denplan care scheme. Virtually all of these patients pay their subscriptions individually without assistance from their employees. The availability of third-party funding schemes has been important in facilitating conversion from NHS to private dentistry during the 1990s and continues to be so. It is important to note, however, that third-party schemes are a relatively small source of funding. Capitation, full indemnity insurance and cash plans combined account for around 10% of general dental practitioners' gross income. Cash paid out of patients' own pockets, in contrast, accounts for approximately 30% and therefore remains by far the dominant mode of private payment. Future growth in the private market would therefore seem to be heavily reliant upon patients being able and willing to pay private prices.

Going hand-in-hand with increased third-party participation in dentistry is the growing involvement of corporate bodies. In July 2005, largely as a result of pressure to comply with European Union competition law, an amendment to the Dentists Act 1984 removed all restrictions on the number of 'bodies corporate', which had previously been held at a steady 28. Since then the corporate dental sector has expanded and in October 2010 it was estimated to account for around 10% of the dentistry market.[32] Any corporate body can now carry out the business of dentistry, provided that it can satisfy the conditions of board membership set out in the amended Act – namely, that the majority of directors of any body corporate must be registered dentists or registered dental care professionals. It is clear that the whole issue of corporate bodies in dentistry is an emotive one, with strong voices both in favour and against. Some dentists feel threatened, raising concerns about the poaching of patients and ancillary staff. While the corporates undoubtedly have the ability to raise considerable capital to establish large new practices, a long-held concern among some members of the profession is that if profits do not accrue, then corners may be cut on materials used and on treatment quality or the range of treatments provided.

The BDA's view on corporate bodies is essentially open-minded – provided that high ethical and clinical standards are maintained and that individual dentists can act at all times in the interest of the patient. This more positive view of corporate bodies currently seems to be carrying the most weight and as such is in favour of the move to abolish present legal restrictions, thus removing at least one obstacle to individuals or groups of dentists gaining the advantages of corporate body status.

It is certainly the proclaimed wish of many of these corporate dental groups to emphasise the personal, continuing relationship of the dentist and patient and so an important task is seen to be the recruitment of dentists with both good clinical skills *and* good communication skills. The corporates have expanded rapidly from a small base and are expected to continue to expand rapidly in the future and continue to influence the rest of the dental profession. In recent times there has been a proliferation of newer, smaller corporates aimed mainly at the NHS market. Some of the larger supermarket chains have also entered the fray, opening up clinics in key locations across the UK. It seems likely that these trends will continue in the future. In some cases they have raised the ante by adopting carefully thought-out strategies in a host of areas already alluded to: visionary leadership; a commitment to quality; a patient-led approach; staff selection, training and motivation; and not least financial control.

Whenever a practice makes the decision to close its doors to NHS patients, it is faced with so many new challenges – deciding on the range of services and treatment options to be provided, managing and motivating staff members, and not least re-evaluating the financial basis of the practice, particularly in terms of pricing and collection policy. Any practice, whatever its size or nature of its funding, and no matter how excellent the treatment provided or how motivated and well-trained the staff, cannot be considered to be genuinely successful unless the management is firmly committed to maintaining its financial health. Excellent practices put in place a carefully considered pricing strategy, as well as establishing comprehensive guidelines in areas such as collection policies and payment methods.

REMOVAL OF ADVERTISING RESTRICTIONS

Until the mid 1970s, virtually all professional service providers such as doctors, dentists, lawyers and accountants were prevented from advertising by restrictions imposed upon them by the various professions' own regulatory bodies. This was a worldwide phenomenon and the primary reasoning behind these restrictions was equally universal and consistent – namely, that such advertising was deemed to be unprofessional and would lower the status of the professions in the eyes of the public. However, by the late 1970s it was clear that, in the United States at least, the professions were coming under increasing pressure to deregulate, paradoxically through public as well as governmental pressure. This move towards deregulation can be traced to the seminal judicial interpretations concerning commercial free speech[34,35] and restraint of trade by professional organisations.[36] These effectively removed any constraints on marketing imposed by a whole range of professional associations and as a result, by 1983, American dentists were allowed to advertise their services freely to the public.

Following the precedent set by the US authorities, a number of other countries have also embraced dental advertising, including the UK, where the earliest discussions in this area stemmed from a Monopolies Commission report looking into the restrictive practices adopted by a variety of professions.[37] The commission found numerous examples that they concluded were against the public interest. Among these were the constraints relating to marketing that, by denial of information concerning individual practitioners and practices, limited consumer choice or made the optimum selection difficult or impossible. The main wave of deregulation began when the British Medical Association declared:

> *Patients are entitled to be given comprehensive, detailed and accurate information about medical services available to them. Doctors working within the National Health Service as opposed to private practice have particular obligations imposed on them by their terms of service by which they must provide both personal, professional and practice information.*[38]

The dental profession quickly followed suit and, by 1988, the only restrictions applied to advertising were those applicable to all advertising – namely, that it be 'truthful, decent and honest'.

The 2012 Office of Fair Trading report[32] drew attention to the fact that many patients were put under pressure by their dentist to sign up to advertised payment plans, commenting that, as a result, these patients are denied the opportunity to make active, informed decisions regarding how they pay for their dental treatment and even what treatment is actually required. The study found that a staggering 82% of dental patients who received a course of dental treatment that incurred a charge did not receive a written treatment plan. Among a raft of suggestions made in the Department of Health's *Review of the Regulation of Cosmetic Interventions*[39] published in 2013 were the following:

- banning free consultations for cosmetic surgery so that people don't feel obliged to go through with surgical procedure
- ensuring consultations are with a medical practitioner and not a sales adviser
- imposing tighter restrictions on advertising including banning two-for-one, time-limited deals and cosmetic surgery as competition prizes.

This report did not target dentistry specifically, but the parallels are obvious.

All this does not mean that advertising is unprofessional but, rather, that the nature and tone is critical and to repeat it should be 'truthful, decent and honest'. Whether or not it is effective is an entirely different matter, since little research has been done to determine if advertising does actually result in greater consumer awareness of dental issues and services and does subsequently lead to increased attendance. You have probably heard the quote about half the money spent on advertising being wasted, you just don't know which half. It has been attributed to everyone from Lord Leverhulme (1851–1925) to John Wanamaker (1838–1922) to Leo Burnett (1891–1971) to David Ogilvy (1911–99). It does not matter who said it or when, because the way advertising money is spent has not changed enough to alter the significance of that statement. It is probably still true. As far as dentistry is concerned, most studies in this area come to the same conclusion; namely, that word of mouth is a far more persuasive influence – primarily for the reason that patients tend to give more credence to the opinions of friends and family than to promotional material put out by the service provider. It has to be remembered that advertising is just one piece of the overall marketing jigsaw and, given that word of mouth is likely to be more effective in persuading consumers, effort and resources would perhaps be better employed in hiring and training staff who possess positive attitudes towards dentistry in general, the practice in particular and, without question, an interest in people as human beings, not just mouths to be fixed. Nevertheless, there is always scope for innovative approaches to marketing and the most effective strategies are by no means always the most expensive. A focused marketing plan comprises a comprehensive and ongoing marketing strategy involving not only obvious promotional strategies but also an understanding that marketing is built around the day-to-day interactions or 'moments of truth' that take place between the practice and its patients.

GLOBALISATION

UK dentists are no longer practising in a vacuum. As far as our profession is concerned, we are no longer an island. Many European Union dentists are now working here and, conversely, many patients are travelling abroad for the perceived cost benefits of having treatment done in places such as eastern Europe and even as far afield as Thailand and the Philippines. Dental laboratories are a major example of this ever-shrinking world. While at one time UK dentists would send their work to the local laboratory, these days they are just as likely to see their work going to set-ups in the Far East or even Africa. The same applies to dental supplies, traditionally provided by large companies in North America and Europe. These businesses are now having to face stiff competition from manufacturers around the world with lower cost structures. Such competition in all these fields is a good thing, provided that high standards are maintained. One thing is for sure and that is such global influence upon the UK market is not going to go away any time soon – rather, it is set to intensify in the years to come.

SUMMARY

It is clear that dentistry in the UK is undergoing the same metamorphosis that has taken place in many other Western cultures. The reaction of entrepreneurs to these changes falls into three groups:
1. those who bury their heads in the sand and refuse to recognise that change is taking place
2. those who allow the changes to happen to them and are tossed and turned by the tide
3. those who recognise that these changes represent a springboard loaded with opportunity for the future.

The rest of this book explores how to treat the current situation not as a threat but as an opportunity. While corporate dentistry probably isn't going to go away, we firmly believe that the successful small business of the future will need to be bespoke and five-star in its outlook – providing a high-quality service to a relatively select group. Of a UK adult population of around 51.4 million, it is estimated that there will be 29.7 million taxpayers in 2012–13. Around 3.8 million of these will pay tax at the higher rate, providing 36.5% of total income tax revenue, and 307 000 taxpayers will pay tax at the additional rate, providing 24.6% of total income tax revenue. As Willie Sutton, the American gangster, said when asked why he robbed banks, 'because that's where the money is', it seems to make sense in business for you to leverage your time and efforts to those people with the greatest disposable income. The trends described in these last few pages interplay with one another to create the modern dental profession and point to the need for practitioners to balance clinical and managerial aspects of their practice. It is apparent that the modern dental practitioner must be able to provide an ethical, appropriate, high-quality service to increasingly sophisticated, knowledgeable and demanding patients, often being held accountable to outside bodies, while at the same time managing an organisation within an increasingly hostile and competitive business environment.

It is against this background that we ask you to consider the first of our eight strategies . . .

REFERENCES

1. National Institute for Health and Care Excellence (NICE). *Prophylaxis against Infective Endocarditis: NICE guideline 64*. London: NICE; 2008.
2. Steele J, O'Sullivan I. *Adult Dental Health Survey 2009*. London: Health and Social Care Information Centre; 2011.
3. General Dental Council. *Compulsory Continuing Professional Development (CPD)*. London: General Dental Council; 2003.
4. General Dental Council. *Guidance on Principles of Management Responsibility*. London: General Dental Council; 2008.
5. Young BDA dentists give their vision of dentistry. *BDA News*. 1999; January: 1.
6. Austin M. Demise of the single handed practitioner. *Br Dent J*. 2013; **214**(5): 218.
7. Hewitt P. *Trust, Assurance and Safety – The Regulation of Health Professionals in the 21st Century* [White Paper]. London: The Stationery Office; 2007.
8. *Revalidation for Dentists: Our proposals*. London: General Dental Council; 2010.
9. http://old.dentistry.co.uk/news/3552-Revalidation-will-slash-dental-patient-numbers
10. Nuffield Foundation. *Education and Training of Personnel Auxiliary to Dentistry*. London: Nuffield Foundation; 1993.
11. *The First Five Years: The undergraduate dental curriculum*. London: General Dental Council; 1997.
12. General Dental Council Dental Auxiliaries Review Group. *Professionals Complementary to Dentistry: A consultation paper*. London: General Dental Council; 1998.

13. British Dental Association. *Direct Access Decision Misguided Says BDA*. Press release. London: British Dental Association; 28 March 2013.
14. General Dental Council. *Standards for Practice*. London: General Dental Council; 2005.
15. General Dental Council. *Standards for the Dental Team*. London: General Dental Council; 2008. Available at: www.gdc-uk.org/Newsandpublications/Publications/Publications/Standards%20for%20the%20Dental%20Team.pdf (accessed 16 November 2013).
16. General Dental Council. *Annual Report and Accounts 2012*. London: General Dental Council; 2012.
17. Dell Computer Company advertisement
18. Dawe T. Can you trust your dentist? *Reader's Digest*. 1998; **152**(January): 50–7.
19. McGrath C, Bedi R. Population based norming of the UK oral health related quality of life measurement (OHQoL-UK). *Br Dent J*. 2002; **193**(9): 521–4.
20. Merrick R. CQC measures 'challenging' for dentists. *Dentistry*. 27 February 2013.
21. British Dental Association. *CQC Failings Laid Bare by Report Says BDA*. Press release. London: British Dental Association; 14 September 2011.
22. Department of Health and Social Security. *Report of the Committee of Inquiry into Unnecessary Dental Treatment*. London: Her Majesty's Stationery Office; 1986.
23. Cooper CL, Watts J, Kelly M. Job satisfaction, mental health, and job stressors among general dental practitioners in the UK. *Br Dent J*. 1987; **162**(2): 77–81.
24. Waddington TJ. New stressors for GDPs in the past 10 years. *Br Dent J*. 1997; **182**(3): 82–3.
25. House of Commons Health Committee. *Report on the Dental Services*. London: Her Majesty's Stationery Office; 1993.
26. Bloomfield SK. *Fundamental Review of Dental Remuneration*. London: Her Majesty's Stationery Office; 1992.
27. Department of Health. *NHS Dentistry: Options for change*. London: 2002.
28. Department of Health. *Standard General Dental Services (GDS) Contract (Revised)*. London: 2005.
29. Hall C. Thousands left without access to NHS dentists. *Daily Telegraph*. 29 March 2007.
30. House of Commons Health Committee. *Dental Services: Fifth Report of Session 2007–08*. London: The Stationery Office; 2008.
31. Steele J, Rooney E, Clarke J, *et al*. *NHS Dental Services in England*. London: Department of Health; 2009.
32. Office of Fair Trading (OFT). *Dentistry: An OFT market study*. London: OFT; 2012.
33. Laing & Buisson. *Dentistry UK Market Report 2011*. 3rd ed. London: Laing & Buisson; 2011.
34. Virginia State Board of Pharmacy v. Virginia Citizens' Consumer Council 425 US 748, 1976.
35. Bates v. State Bar of Arizona 433 US 350, 1977.
36. Goldfarb v. Virginia State Bar 421 US 773, 1975.
37. Monopolies Commission. *Professional Services: A report on the general effect on the public interest of certain restrictive practices so far as they prevail in relation to the supply of professional services*. London: Her Majesty's Stationery Office; 1970.
38. British Medical Association. *Guidelines to Doctors on Advertising*. London: British Medical Association; 1991.
39. Keogh B. *Review of the Regulation of Cosmetic Interventions*. London: Department of Health; 2013.

CHAPTER TWO

Strategy 1: Construct a powerful three-year vision

Good business leaders create a vision, articulate the vision, passionately own the vision, and relentlessly drive it to completion.

Jack Welch, former CEO of General Electric

Who is the most important person in your practice? These days dentists are almost programmed to respond with . . . 'the patient', and of course this answer makes a lot of sense, doesn't it? After all, how often are you told that 'the customer is king' or that 'the customer always knows best'? However, while it might seem somewhat contrary to say so, in truth, the most important person in the practice is *you*. While it is of course true that the practice should ultimately focus on its clientele (they are, after all, the source of all your income), you are nevertheless the person whose responsibility it is to set that focus, to establish the fundamental nature of the practice and to bring on board, shape and mould like-minded team members. If you aren't going to do these things, who is? Therefore, we believe that you are, without doubt, the most important person in your practice. Without your vision, inspiration and guidance your business won't go very far – there simply won't be many customers to please. The first step, therefore, on the road to creating a practice that everyone wants to visit is to gain clarity of purpose by constructing a vision of where you are heading, both personally and professionally over short-, medium- and long-term time frames. To do so you need to understand yourself and what drives you. You need to understand your own deep-seated values because for a vision to be meaningful and, importantly, *effective*, it must be a true reflection of your hopes and aspirations and it must be in harmony with what you believe and hold to be true about yourself.

This may all seem a bit wishy-washy, or vague even, especially when you are champing at the bit to get on and mobilise your practice. After all, isn't it true that as a dentist you are trained to solve complex technical problems, without agonising too much over the deeper philosophical meaning behind what you do? If you actually believe this, then you are selling yourself seriously short.

Without giving due consideration to the deep-seated, fundamental beliefs that make you tick, you will never build a practice in which you and your staff enjoy working, one that patients love to visit and one that will give you the financial rewards you desire. A few years ago I (PN) spoke on the subject of 'core values' at a young dentists' conference held in Blackpool one cold weekend in November. At the end of my talk one young man, recently graduated, came up to me and congratulated me on my ability to spin out for one hour a subject that he felt could have been covered in 10 minutes. Needless to say I felt quite dejected. Then another, older, dentist came over and said that when he had just graduated he would have thought the same as the first dentist and would have headed off to find the bar. However, now he was a bit more mature and was actually running his own practice and trying, with some difficulty, to get his team to tune into his own ideas, he could see how fundamentally important it was to identify one's own core values, articulate them and use them as the basis of where he and his practice were heading. Feeling vindicated, I too headed off to the bar.

Writing in *The E-Myth Revisited*, Michael Gerber[1] asks you to consider the following questions: 'What do I value most?' 'What kind of life do I want?' 'What do I want my life to look like, to feel like?' 'Who do I wish to be?' These are fundamental questions, the answers to which should be seen as the basic blueprint for how you manage your life. However you answer them, it is very likely that your business, your practice, is going to be as major a component of that blueprint as your personal life. With this in mind, what is your vision?

YOUR THREE-YEAR VISION

Do you have an inspiring and compelling vision of the future? For your business? For your personal life? This might be a lot for people to take on board, but here's the truth:

> You CAN design the perfect life and you CAN design the perfect business and you CAN have it.

A big question: If we were meeting here in three years' time, and looking back over the previous 36 months, what would have to have happened to you both personally and professionally for you to be satisfied with your progress?

1.

2.

3.

4.

5.

6.

7.

Note: remember your goals can relate to work, financial, family, physical, social, intellectual or spiritual matters.

When you have your vision, share it with your business associates and support team. Let them know what your intentions are and where the business is going. Have them understand that they are all part of the process and that there will be compensation for them as they work towards its success. The three-year vision, along with other exercises we will ask you to work on, is a living, breathing document. In other words, it will be constantly changing and you will want to refer to it every day in some form or another. Think of it in terms of being a 1000-day rolling vision that changes every 24 hours.

Writing down your three-year vision will help you answer the type of questions posed by Michael Gerber[1]:

> With no clear picture of how you wish your life to be, how on earth can you begin to live it? How would you know what first step to take? How would you measure your progress? How would you know where you were, how far you had gone and how much farther you had yet to go?

Successful people, great people, have a vision of their lives, a vision that they endeavour to match every day. They don't let life simply happen to them, passively waiting to see what will happen to them next. They are proactive in creating the life that they want. Great people look at their life as it is, compare that with the vision they have set themselves and see what needs to be done to make up the difference. This is the difference between what Gerber and others describe as living intentionally and existing by accident. So what would you like to be doing three months from now? Two years from now? Ten years from now? What would you like to learn during your life – spiritually, physically, financially, technically, intellectually? How much money will you need to do the things you wish to do? When will you need this money? The answers to these questions set the standards against which you can judge your progress. Without them your life will drift along without direction.

Since people behave according to the nature and strength of their basic core values, then the way you, your staff and your patients interact is ultimately dependent upon those core values. While such values cannot easily be altered or manipulated, by understanding them it is possible to build teams of people who, by and large, share the same underlying beliefs. As will be shown later, such teams tend to be stronger, more unified, more highly motivated and ultimately more productive than groups of people who do not.

WHAT ARE YOUR VALUES?

Your life and, as we will see in a moment, your business will proceed much more smoothly when aligned with your core values. Take the time to think carefully about the following questions and answer them as honestly and as specifically as possible. Your answers will help you to determine those things that are of key importance in your life.

If you were to do one thing in your personal life that would have the most impact, what would that one thing be?

What are the tangible and intangible things that you would most like to have in life?

What would you most like to do with your life?

What kind of person would you most like to be?

DETERMINING YOUR KEY VALUES

Look back over your life and try to recall times when you felt completely yourself – when you felt alive, excited, fulfilled and full of natural energy. Was it when you used to draw and paint as a child? If so, it's possible that 'creativity' is an important value for you. Perhaps it was when you travelled to some exotic part of the world, or decided to take up hang-gliding or rock climbing? If so, then maybe one of your key values would be 'adventure'.

What are your priorities? If one of your top priorities is spending time with your spouse and children, then one of your key values might be 'family'. As you identify your values, it's a good idea to define them. By clarifying your values, they become more real to you. Also, your definition may be very different from someone else's. For example, to you, 'professionalism' might mean delivering a consistently five-star service, whereas for someone else it might be always showing up on time for appointments. When you write your personal definitions be sure to use positive statements such as 'I am', 'I do', 'I will'.

Please list your key values below along with clarifying statements for each one. A list of some more common values is shown in the column on the right. You may want to choose some of these and/or add your own, unique values.

Value 1:
Personal definition

Value 2:
Personal definition

Value 3:
Personal definition

and so on . . .

Accomplishment
Adventure
Authenticity
Balance
Beauty
Career
Communication
Community
Compassion
Connecting
Courage
Creativity
Education
Excellence
Family
Fitness
Freedom
Fun
Gratitude
Happiness
Helping others
Honesty
Integrity
Laughter
Learning
Love
Loyalty
Making a difference
Patience
Peace
Respect
Self-expression
Serenity
Spirituality
Taking care of myself
Teamwork
Winning

THE LINK BETWEEN CORE VALUES AND BUSINESS SUCCESS

The collective core values of an organisation constitute the 'climate' or 'culture' of that organisation – a potpourri of deep-set values, ideals, attitudes, beliefs and behaviours that influence how people work together. These core values are, or should be, an organisation's essential and enduring tenets – a small set of general guiding principles, not to be compromised for financial gain or short-term expediency. This applies just as much to a dental practice as it does to a large multinational organisation, and it is just as crucial to the practice's long-term viability and success. There is a growing acceptance in the business world that firms holding a strong set of values tend to be the most successful and tend to stay around the longest. Without core values clearly and solidly established at the heart of the dental practice, performance will always be limited.[2] In their seminal book on corporate governance, *Built to Last*, James Collins and Jerry Porras[3] point to clear evidence that if your only value is making money, then this isn't going to be enough to get and keep the best people and to sustain success over the long term. They also stress that visionary organisations don't merely declare an ideology, they also:

- more thoroughly indoctrinate employees into a core ideology than comparison companies, creating cultures so strong that they are almost cult-like around that ideology
- more carefully nurture and select staff based on fit with a core ideology than the comparison companies
- attain more consistent alignment with a core ideology – in such aspects as goals, strategy, tactics and organisation design – than the comparison companies.

It is easy to see why a dental practice with clearly defined values would be more successful if one considers the following sequence of events:

- as we will show you in Strategy 5 (Deliver world-class customer service) of this book, your patients evaluate dental practices more on the 'softer' aspects of care (aspects they do understand and feel competent to evaluate), than on the 'hard' technical skills of the dentist (which they feel ill-equipped to evaluate); accordingly . . .
- everyone in the practice, not just the dentist, is included in the patient's overall evaluation as well as every 'transaction' conducted with the practice; hence it follows that . . .
- a team comprising highly motivated staff members dedicated towards providing the best in customer care is likely to be evaluated positively by the patient. Such a team is far more likely to be achieved when . . .

- core values and ideologies are clearly stated, staff feel in tune with these values and feel highly motivated to act upon them.

INCORPORATING YOUR VALUES INTO YOUR PRACTICE

In *Priorities, Practice and Ethics in Small Firms,* a report compiled for the Institute of Business Ethics, Laura Spence[4] states that many owners of small firms are guided by strong principles even though they are rarely formalised into any kind of enforceable code of practice. She recommends 10 practical rules for good business conduct, as shown in Box 2.1.

BOX 2.1 Ten practical rules for good business conduct[4]

1 Establish your core business values and stick to them or your reputation will suffer.
2 Welfare and motivation of your staff are critical to your success.
3 If you need partners make sure they share your vision and values.
4 Work at your relations with customers; they neither start nor stop when the sale is made.
5 Don't knock your competitors.
6 Stick to your agreed terms of payment.
7 Record all financial transactions in your books.
8 Find at least one way of supporting communities in which you operate.
9 If you are doubtful about an ethical issue in your business, take advice.

and last, but not least . . .

10 Remember that the owner-manager's business behaviour will be taken as the role model by staff.

It would be difficult to find anything contained in this list that is not relevant to dental practice. Indeed, without necessarily being aware of the fact, most dentists are already behaving in accordance with these guidelines! Problems eventually arise when people working in a practice hold fundamentally different values. These can be on just about anything – for example, the value of treatment offered, the way people should be addressed, dress code, and so on. Such 'value gaps' lead to confusion, conflict and tension and inevitably a reduced quality of service.[5]

It is no coincidence that the first rule on this list is concerned with the establishment of core values. This is a crucial first step and one that ultimately underscores everything else that happens in the practice. To illustrate this point, consider the example of a philosophy statement in Box 2.2 that articulates quite clearly the underlying ethos of the practice in question.

BOX 2.2 Philosophy statement

A patient is the most important visitor on our premises.
He is not dependent on us – we are dependent on him.

He is not an outsider in our business – he is part of it.

We are not doing him a favour by serving him – he is doing us a favour by giving us the opportunity to do so.

This is, in effect, a vision statement, a general declaration specifying the fundamental strategy or intent that governs your goals and objectives. A practice vision statement encapsulates your 'reason for being' and enables you to clarify your purpose for yourself, your staff and others who are interested. In order to create your own personal vision statement you must first identify the various roles that you fulfil in your life:

- roles representing the key relationships you have with other people
- roles representing your principal areas of responsibility in life
- roles representing the areas in which you can make a contribution.

STEPS TO IDENTIFYING YOUR KEY ROLES

List each of the roles you play in life – for example, spouse, parent, business owner, friend, community member, sports team member. You may want to combine functions to keep your total number of roles to seven or fewer. Don't forget to include 'myself' as one of the roles. List the people connected with each role – for example, in your role as employer, the key people associated with that role would be your staff.

Finally, write a description of your ideal performance in each role – even if this is not the reality at the moment. For example, using the example of 'parent' you might write:

> *I give my children unlimited love and support. I am always available to take them to important events; I make it safe for them to say anything to me; I encourage honest communication at all times.*

Remember to use positive statements when describing your ideal performance in each role.

Role 1:   *Key people:*

Ideal performance:

Role 2:   *Key people:*

Ideal performance:

Role 3:   *Key people:*

Ideal performance:

and so on . . .

How much time are you spending in each role? Mark on the pie chart the percentage of time you currently spend in each of your roles. Is it enough? Too much?

How much time would you like to spend in each area?

If you could wave a realistic magic wand, how would you like the chart to look?

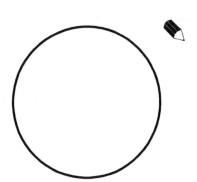

Example

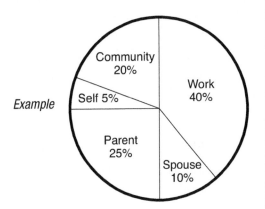

Mark the chart again, this time with percentages relating to the amount of time you would ideally like to be devoting to each of your roles.

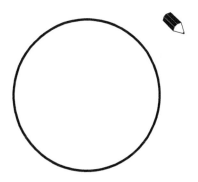

What needs to change for this to happen?

YOUR MISSION STATEMENT

You are now almost ready to construct your own personal and professional mission statements. Having a mission helps you to focus the direction of your goals. It is important to realise that there is no such thing as a ready-made off-the-shelf philosophy statement, and it has to be said that business mission statements in particular have come in for considerable criticism in recent years, the problem being their tendency to create hollow values. A glaring example of this occurred recently with the collapse of the giant US energy company Enron. This particular company's 2001 annual report ironically centred on and stressed core values of 'communication, respect, integrity, and excellence' – could anything have ever been further from the truth! Writing in the *Harvard Business Review*, Patrick Lencioni[6] notes that most value statements are bland, toothless or just plain dishonest and, far from being harmless, they are often highly destructive. Empty value statements, espoused but not practised by management personified by an attitude of 'care for your customers – or else!' alienate customers, create cynical and dispirited employees, and undermine managerial credibility.

CONSTRUCT YOUR MISSION STATEMENT

Athletes have an expression they call 'the zone'. When they are in the zone they feel absolutely wonderful – it's going so well they don't even know they are doing it. You are in the flow and it seems as if whatever you are doing requires no effort. You are happy. You are fulfilled. It is going well. You are centred.

Keep this in mind when you answer these questions:

What are your greatest moments of happiness and fulfilment?

What are the activities of most worth in your professional life?

What are the activities of most worth in your personal life?

What talents/capabilities do you have?

How would you like to best contribute to the world?

Imagine you have lived a fulfilling, rewarding life and it is now your 80th birthday.

Your friends, family, professional colleagues and those from the community have gathered to celebrate with you and pay you tribute. What would you like them to say?

List each of your roles and imagine a person paying tribute to you in each of those roles. Then write down what you would like each of them to say.

Role 1:   *Person paying tribute:*

Role 2:   *Person paying tribute:*

and so on . . .

How close are you *now* to fulfilling these tributes?

Use the information and insights you've gleaned from this and the previous exercises to construct your personal and professional mission statements. You might find it useful to use the template from Stephen Covey *et al.*'s book *First Things First* when doing this exercise.[7] You answer questions and your mission statement is compiled automatically and emailed to you.

For any mission statement to be effective, no one but yourself can come up with it, and as far as your professional mission statement is concerned no one but yourself can enunciate those basic creeds that will be central to how you run your practice. When we say 'yourself' we mean you and your staff – your team *must* feel that they are playing a central part in this process. If they do not believe that the statement reflects their feelings, do not feel that they too 'own' the statement then it will become as hollow as all the others. You must create a consuming vision for your practice and share this with your team so that they are fully briefed on where the practice is heading in the future, and can be part of the process. Equally, you must show your patients you have a positive overview of the way your practice is progressing. Your enthusiasm will generate all-important trust and confidence.

Do not fall into the trap of using the core values of other practices, even successful ones. Core ideology does not come from mimicking the values of others and it does not come from a sterile intellectual exercise of 'calculating' what values would be most pragmatic, most popular or most profitable. When articulating core ideology, the key step is to capture what is authentically believed, not what others state as their values or what the outside world thinks the ideology should be.

YOUR VISION IS YOUR BRAND

If you were asked to define, in very basic terms, what your patients, even potential patients, think of you and your practice, how they view you, you might use phrases such as:

- *'what they feel after they have been to see us'*
- *'how they like us as people'*
- *'what they feel about the services we offer'*.

In other words, you would talk about those perceptions and emotions that describe the experience related to 'doing business' with you, which is one way of describing a 'brand'. While many dentists fight the idea of branding, protesting that 'I am a professional, the word branding is totally inappropriate for what I do', they would be foolish to deny that some perception, however ill-defined, of the dentist and his or her practice is nevertheless fermenting away in the subconscious mind of each and every one of his or her clients. This notion is built upon the many, or few, interactions the patient has had with the practice in general and the dentist in particular – in other words, the relationship between the buyer and the seller. In one of the most famous books on the subject of customer service ever written, *Moments of Truth*, former Scandinavian Airlines

System CEO Jan Carlzon[8] used these terms to describe such interactions and said that the whole relationship between provider and consumer hinged on how these exchanges were handled. Branding is not about superficial design or packaging. At its most fundamental level it is a way of characterising a relationship built upon a direct connection between mutually compatible value systems. David McNally and Karl Speak[9] explain just what this means in their excellent book *Be Your Own Brand* (*see* Box 2.3).

BOX 2.3 Definitions of brand[9]

- Brand is how businesses tell customers what to expect. Things can change rapidly in the business world, and customers are more comfortable if they know what to expect.
- Brand is a familiar bridge across which businesses and their customers conduct transactions that lead to long-term and mutually beneficial relationships.
- Brand is the embodiment of what businesses and their customers value, the means through which businesses are given credit for the quality they represent and deliver.

A business' brand is a reflection of who the owners are and what they believe, which is visibly expressed by what they do and how they do it. The image of that brand is a perception held in someone else's mind. As that perception evolves and sharpens through repeated contacts (moments of truth), a brand relationship takes form. It should be clear now, then, that every practice already has a brand – a reflection of what patients think of it. The thing is, only a tiny proportion of the dentists who own those practices are aware of this fact.

Good brands are powerful things. People tend to stick with them. When a particular perception or emotion is fixed in someone's mind then it takes a lot to change or shift it, especially when the brand is highly personalised – as, for example, in the relationship between a dentist and a patient. The resilience of this attachment to a perception of someone or something means that one is likely to be forgiven the odd transgression or failure to fulfil an occasional promise – assuming, of course, that this one-off aberration is just that and doesn't become a routine happening. Likewise, deliver more than someone expects and the relationship is strengthened further. McNally and Speak[9] say that brands start to become strong when you decide what you believe in and then commit yourself to acting on those beliefs. Your brand of dentistry is a reflection of those ideas and values that are distinctively you. This is the only substance upon which a truly lasting relationship can be built.

FINALLY . . .

In both your business and personal life, every now and again there will be one of those days when everything goes wrong; it seems as if everything and everyone is against you and nothing will ever go right again. The faith you have in your core values can be seriously strained. What mechanisms do you have in place for when this happens? Here are some ideas:

- talk to a trusted friend or family member
- make a 'Feel-Good Folder' full of testimonial letters
- compile a scrapbook of the achievements in your life
- read your personal vision statement to remind you of who you are and what is really important in your life. Work out what you are tolerating . . .

WHAT AM I TOLERATING?*

We humans have learned how to tolerate a lot! We put up with, accept, take on and are dragged down by other people's behaviour, situations, unmet needs, crossed boundaries, incompletion, frustrations, problems and even our own behaviour.

You are putting up with more than you think. Take a couple of minutes to write down all the things you sense you are tolerating. As you think of more items, add them to your list.

Just becoming aware of and articulating these intolerations will bring them to the forefront of your mind and you will naturally start handling, eliminating, fixing, growing through and resolving them. You may choose to write down any action you intend to take to resolve the toleration. Some common tolerations are shown in the column on the right.

Toleration	Action
1.	
2.	
3.	
4.	
5.	
6.	
7.	
8.	
9.	
10.	
11.	

* Based on the work of Thomas J Leonard and the coaches at Coach University (www.coachu.com).

Work
Environment
Colleagues
Staff
Clients
Suppliers
Holidays
Working conditions
Procedures
Requirements
Hours
Filing

Family and friends
Spouse/partner
Children
Relatives
Close friends
Social acquaintances
Neighbours

Home
Location
Layout
Cleanliness
Décor
Comfort
Lighting
Storage
Garden
Noise

Yourself
Vitality/energy
Weight
Clothes
Stress
Exercise
Boundaries
Self-esteem
Addictions
Fulfilment
Emotions
Work/play
Anger

Money/credit card debt
Mortgage
Tax
Investments
Insurance
Cash flow
Income

Equipment/appliances
Car
Computer
Home electricals

REFERENCES

1. Gerber M. *The E-Myth Revisited*. New York, NY: Harper Collins; 1995.
2. Cooper MB. Core values and practice success. *J Am Dent Assoc*. 2008; **139**(10): 1405–7.
3. Collins J, Porras J. *Built to Last: Successful habits of visionary companies*. 3rd ed. London: Random House; 2005.
4. Spence L. *Priorities, Practice and Ethics in Small Firms*. London: Institute of Business Ethics; 2000.
5. Newsome PRH, Wolfe IS. Value gaps in dental practice: understanding how differences in core values can adversely affect the practice. *J Am Dent Assoc*. 2003; **134**(11): 1500–4.
6. Lencioni P. Make your values mean something. *Harv Bus Rev*. 2002; **80**(7): 113–17.
7. Covey S, Merrill AR, Merrill RR. *First Things First*. New York, NY: Simon & Schuster; 1999.
8. Carlzon J. *Moments of Truth*. Cambridge, MA: Ballinger; 1989.
9. McNally D, Speak K. *Be Your Own Brand*. San Francisco, CA: Berrett-Koehler; 2003.

FURTHER READING

- Canfield J. Hansen MV, Hewitt L *The Power of Focus*. Deerfield Beach, FL: Health Communications; 2001.
- Covey S. *The 7 Habits of Highly Effective People*. London: Simon & Schuster; 2004.
- Ditzler J. *Your Best Year Yet!* New York. Warner; 2000.
- Gallway WT. *The Inner Game of Work*. London: Random House; 1999.
- Gaskell C. *Transform Your Life*. London: Thorsons Publishing; 2001.
- Newsome P. *The Patient-Centred Dental Practice: A practical guide to customer care*. London: BDJ Books; 2001.

CHAPTER THREE

Strategy 2: Plan the time to plan

Baldrick, you wouldn't recognise a cunning plan if it painted itself purple and danced naked on top of a harpsichord singing 'Cunning plans are here again'.

Ebenezer Blackadder

This strategy is a crucial step in the development of your business success and one that you disregard at your peril. This is where you take time to work *on* your business rather than *in* your business. Unfortunately, most dentists are either unwilling or unable to do this as a matter of routine even though most dentists tend to be most dissatisfied with issues related to practice management ('the business side of my practice is a shambles'), quality of life (in terms of family life, day-to-day interactions with others, friendships, and so on), 'professional time' (e.g. time to keep abreast of advances, time to improve clinical skills, time to devote to patients' needs, and time for professional contacts with colleagues) and, finally, 'personal time' (time available for leisure activities).[1] Back in the 1980s, Cary Cooper and colleagues[2] found that aside from specific medical emergencies, two of the principal sources of stress for practising dentists were running behind schedule and constant time pressures, and that both of these appeared to result in higher levels of physical and mental ill health. These studies suggest that most dentists don't have strategies in place for planning and ordering their vision, their medium- and long-term goals and their day-to-day activities. As we have said before, dentists are trained to act as dentists and when they find that practice is more than that, many start to struggle to make sense of it all.

Dan Sullivan,[3] a Toronto-based strategic coach, asks us to imagine that we are only allowed to have three types of day in our lives:

- free days
- focus days
- buffer days.

FREE DAY = DAY OFF

These are the days on which you rest, recuperate, recharge and reconnect with yourself and with those people that matter outside of work. It is a day when you fulfil your roles as 'self', a family member, a friend, and so forth. Don't address yourself in any way, shape or form to your obligations at work. On free days you are not doing further education, not popping into the office, not checking emails, not doing the business newsletter or the books on the laptop at the kitchen table. There is no work in the boot of your car!

FOCUS DAY = FOCUSED ON GETTING RESULTS

These are the days when you are concentrating on doing whatever you get paid for. You are seeing patients, dealing with clients, selling your product, networking. You are focused on results – doing whatever it is that you are naturally gifted at.

BUFFER DAY = ALL THE OTHER STUFF ASSOCIATED WITH BEING IN BUSINESS

These are the days when you deal with all the other 'stuff' – admin, reading, fixing shelves, business/personal budgets, correspondence, research. How many do you need per week to keep the business rolling? Typically half a day per week should be enough. Explain to your team that you are not to be disturbed if you need to concentrate. Say *no*. Close the door. Think of these as future profit days.

HOW TO PLAN THE TIME TO PLAN

- Plan and book your free, focus and buffer days up to 18 months in advance.
- Buy a diary for this/next year – or get a wall planner – whatever works for you.
- Devise a system to colour-code your diary – use different colours for the three different types of day.
- Decide which weeks you will work and which will be *off*. Colour these on your wall planner and in your diary. Try to avoid taking Friday as your day off. They will find you – wherever you hide! Mondays work much better.
- Some days may be divided into focus and buffer days.
- Make sure that you take entire days for your free days.

Action steps	Target date	Completed
Buy diary or wall planner for this/next year		
Decide on free, focus, buffer days		
Colour-code diary/wall planner		
Comments		

We suggest that you schedule the regular meetings as shown in Table 3.1.

TABLE 3.1 Meetings, bloody meetings!

Frequency	Duration	Description
Daily	20 minutes	Prioritised 'to do' lists
Weekly	1–2 hours	Team meeting: shared status reports
Monthly (includes one weekly)	½ to 1 day	Team meeting: shared status report and 30-day action plan
Quarterly (includes one monthly)	2 days	Workshop then shared status reports and 30-day + 90-day goals
Annually (includes one monthly/quarterly)	2–3 days	Workshop/retreat then shared status reports and 30-day + 90-day goals + annual goals
Total	13–26 days	= 5%–10% of working hours

MONTHLY STRATEGIC PLANNING MEETINGS

What exactly do we mean by strategic planning? What images, for example, does the word *strategy* conjure up in your mind? Wellington outfoxing Napoleon at the Battle of Waterloo? Richard Branson taking on his arch-rival British Airways in the early days of Virgin Atlantic? Or perhaps, the Red Bull Formula One team masterminding yet another Grand Prix victory? What it probably doesn't bring to mind is your own everyday life in dental practice. For one thing, it probably seems too grand a concept, something that doesn't quite fit easily into your own scheme of things. While there is no question where the word comes from (*stratagem*, which can be roughly translated as the 'art of the general'), management experts can't always agree on what exactly it means. Indeed, the authors of the first textbook on marketing strategy decided not to define the term at all because it was too difficult. While you are clearly not alone then in being puzzled by all of this, let's not get too bogged down in theory and semantics. For your purposes your strategy describes how you, as practice leader, would like your practice to go in the future, how you plan to get there and, crucially, how you intend to implement that plan. We have hopefully convinced you in Strategy 1 that, with few exceptions, you would not make a journey without having some notion of where you were heading, and it similarly makes even less sense to allow your business to wander aimlessly into the future without any thought being given to where you want it to go.

You might argue that the business of dentistry is relatively straightforward and only basic common sense is required. Anything other than the most rudimentary planning is superfluous. Our customers know all too well what we offer, and if luck would have it and more of them turn up to take advantage of our services, then we can simply expand. The only advanced planning really needed is ordering supplies and fixing the date of the Christmas party! The flaws in this argument are painfully obvious. For one thing, do existing patients and, more significantly, potential ones really know what you are able to offer them in terms of dentistry enhancing their lives? Maybe they do know we can get them out of pain and fill in holes and gaps between their teeth, but do they really know about and understand all the fantastic options that are open to them nowadays? This is all about adding value to what you do. Adding value means making all your clients aware of *all* the products and services you offer – all the ways that you can help them. This is because consumers label us with expertise in the first thing they buy from us – and often miss the point that we can do lots of other things. For dentists this means escape from the 'drill, fill, bill' mentality towards a view of the complete range of treatment options on offer. If they do, and let's face it the amount of information available to the public is increasing all the time, are you and your staff ready, willing and able to meet the demand for these newer types of treatment?

MAKE THE TIME FOR DAILY STRATEGIC PLANNING

Try to find 15–30 minutes every day to switch everything off, find a sanctuary, close the door and allow yourself the time to think and plan. Do *not* allow yourself to be interrupted. Reflect on what you are hoping to achieve that day – or the following day/week/month, and so on. Do this at a time when you are fresh – that is, not tired, whether you are a morning, midday, evening or late-night person. This is primarily the time when you organise your 'to do' list for the day ahead. Whether you use a personal organiser, a computer, a tablet or your mobile phone, the rules are the same:

- make a list
- ABC the list
- prioritise the As, Bs and Cs
- do the As first!

Weekly reflections

Take some time, each week, to reflect upon the various 'roles' that you decided you filled in Strategy 1. Consider and write down what would have to happen in the following week for you to have the most positive impact in each of these roles.

Role 1:

Role 2:

and so on . . .

We suggest that you hold strategy planning meetings one half-day (three hours) every month. Ideally, your practice manager or equivalent should chair the meeting. A suggested agenda for monthly strategic planning meetings is provided here. To make sure the meetings are productive and valuable, and to keep you focused, follow these three simple steps as you discuss each item:

Consider – Decide – Act.

Finance

- Review of management accounts for last month
- Review of management accounts for the year to date
- Course corrections required
- Current cash flow situation
- Action needed to accelerate cash flow
- Review of current pricing strategy

Sales

- Review of sales versus target for the previous month
- Review of sales versus target for the year to date
- Analysis of sales by product/service
- Analysis of sales by customer grade/group
- Review of current selling skills within team
- Review of common objections from customers – and the answers
- Role-play sessions scheduled
- Review of new products/services and how they will be sold

Marketing

- Review of customer grading
- Review of added-value methods
- Review of newsletter
- Review of referral system
- Review of networking activity
- Review of strategic alliances
- Review of documentation and corporate image
- Review of marginal marketing techniques
- Review of publishing and public relations activity

Resources

- Review of existing environment and facilities
- Review of additional facilities required
- Revisions to budgets and targets as a result of purchasing decisions

Personnel

- Review of team performance (the 'helium culture' – *see* Strategy 4, page 77)
- Review of individual performance
- Review of discretionary bonus system year to date
- Team development

- Team training
- Review of personal progress interview system (*see* Strategy 4, page 77)

STRATEGIC PLANNING MEETINGS: PROGRESS CHART

You should keep track of your progress on this chart.

Month of meeting   **Key insights or points raised**

January

February

. . . and so on

STRATEGIC PLANNING MEETINGS: FOLLOW-UP AND GOALS

After each meeting complete the following chart, distribute copies of it to key personnel and use it to track progress within the practice. Bear in mind the words of Harry Beckwith: 'There is no performance without accountability, there is no accountability without measurement'.[4]

		Goals set	**Person responsible**	**Date of meeting** **Target dates**	**Done**
Finance					
Sales					
Marketing					
Resources					
Personnel					

SOME USEFUL DEFINITIONS

We have found it useful to make a distinction between the following:

- three-year vision
- one-year plan
- 90-day action
- monthly management
- weekly reflection
- daily tasks.

Three-year vision

This is the ultimate destination, measured by reference to the *roles* that you have chosen for yourself (*see* Strategy 1, page 23). This is the 'school essay' that describes the life you would like to be living, professionally and personally, in three years' time. Remember to write in pencil – you are allowed to change it continuously.

One-year plan

What has to have happened in one year's time, for you to be on track for the vision? This is a list of SMART goals – specific, measurable, action-oriented, realistic, and time- and resource-constrained (*see* Box 3.1). Again this is compiled by reference to your *roles*.

BOX 3.1 Writing SMART goal statements

A goal statement formalises:

- *what* is to be accomplished
- *who* will be involved
- *when* the activity will be completed
- *how much* cost and resources will be used.

The SMART approach to goal writing ensures that all these elements are included:

- *Specific* means detailed, particular or focused. A goal is specific when everyone knows exactly what is to be achieved and accomplished.
- *Measurable* goals are quantifiable and provide a standard for comparison, the means to an end, a specific result.
- *Action-oriented* means that the goal statements indicate an activity, a performance or something that produces results.
- *Realistic* goals are practical, achievable and possible. Goals must motivate people to improve and to reach for attainable ends.
- *Time- and resource-constrained* means scheduled, regulated by time and resources to be expended, a deadline.

Sounds simple doesn't it? So let's look at one particular situation to see what can happen. Let's suppose that you are getting a bit concerned about the amount of time that your surgery assistant is taking to clean up between patients. Admittedly, this isn't perhaps something you would have in mind when you are putting together your one-year plan, but it does serve to illustrate the mechanics (and some of the pitfalls) of the process.

Be specific

Being specific means spelling out the details of the goal. For example, setting a goal for your surgery assistant to 'make better use of time' is too general for a goal statement because it does not provide any specific information about what is to be accomplished. On the other hand, 'reduce the time taken to ready the surgery for the next patient' specifies the desired improvement and leaves little doubt about what is to be achieved.

Be measurable

In this particular example, 'reduce the time taken to ready the surgery for the next patient' is a specific statement, but to be measurable it needs the addition of, say, '. . . to two minutes'.

Be action-oriented

In the statement 'reduce the time taken to ready the surgery for the next patient to two minutes', 'the verb 'reduce' indicates that the expected result is to lower the turnover time from the existing level to a more desirable level.

Be realistic

The goal *'reduce the time taken to ready the surgery for the next patient to two minutes'* is possible and achievable (i.e. realistic) only if the time taken at the moment is, say, three minutes. If the time taken currently is around five minutes, then two minutes may not be realistic.

Be time- and resource-constrained

People generally put off doing things if no deadline is set, because human nature always finds something else to do that has a higher priority. For example, 'by the end of March' is more specific than '. . . soon'. Some goals are easily achieved when money and resources are unlimited. For example, one way of achieving the goal of reducing the surgery turnaround time to two minutes would be to employ an extra surgery assistant. In the real world, however, money and resources are constraints that must be considered. Dental practice is clearly, no different in that respect from any other business.

So there we are, a clearly defined, easily achievable goal – all that is left for you to do now is tell your dental surgery assistant of your plans, right? Well not quite! Your dental surgery assistant can easily see a goal such as this as being somewhat threatening, and understandably so: *'OK Sheila, it's taking you far too long to clean up the surgery between patients and I have decided that you must cut that time by 30% by the end of March.'* The result is probably not at all what you originally envisaged. At best Sheila starts to sulk, tells everyone that you are a slave-driver and at worst, decides she doesn't like working there anymore and simply doesn't turn up for work one day. Your great plan to shave a few minutes off your turnaround time doesn't sound too clever now, does it? You may even begin to question whether the goal was worth pursuing at all. If you do decide that the time between patients has to be cut and, in most cases, you really have to wonder whether those extra couple of minutes is worth fretting over, then how you communicate the need for change to your staff is vital and a true test of your leadership style. As the old saying goes, *Be careful of what you wish for, you might just get it!*

90-day action

What are the goals you need to set in the next 90 days to move you towards your plan? Write them down and share them with your partner, team, family and advisor.[5] Put them somewhere where you will see them regularly.

---

21 GOALS TO REACH IN THE NEXT 90 DAYS

                                                            Start Date
                                                            Finish Date

What are the goals you most want to set for yourself over the next 90 days? Please select those goals that you really want, not the ones you should, could, ought to or might want. Give some serious thought to setting both your professional and personal goals. When you have set the right goals for yourself, you should feel excited, a little nervous, ready and willing to go for it!

Don't choose the goals you have historically chosen but never reached, unless you're in a much better position to reach them now.

Business

1.

2.

3.

Financial

1.

2.

3.

Family

1.

2.

3.

Social

1.

2.

3.

Physical

1.

2.

3.

Intellectual

1.

2.

3.

Spiritual

1.

2.

3.

Monthly management

This is your personal and professional 'board meeting' where you review finance, sales, marketing, resources and personnel. It's your chance to take a positional reading and make course corrections. Like a sailing vessel, you tack towards your destination.

Weekly reflection

Organise a time, once a week, where you find a sanctuary and reflect upon the whole process. Ask yourself two questions: first, what were your key achievements in the last week, and second, what are your key achievements for the coming week – all measured by reference to *roles*. Remember, you desire steady progress, not perfection, in all areas of your life.

Daily tasks

This is the time management bit – make a list of all you have to do today. ABC the list; do the As first.

There is a clear link between the short-, medium- and long-term in your life. They integrate to a whole picture. Repeat this process every day, week, quarter, year and you will constantly evolve into a more advanced version of you.

THE PLANNING PROCESS IN ACTION

Putting all of these ideas together, consider the following case study (names and locations have been changed for obvious reasons) – a prime example of how things can end up when planning is poorly managed.

BOX 3.2 Case study

Roger Bell BDS ran a busy, single-handed NHS practice in the centre of a small market town. A few days earlier he had attended a lecture given by a prominent dentist from London on the subject of home tooth whitening. The lecturer told his audience that as a result of magazine articles, information on the internet and growing word of mouth, more and more patients in the future would be demanding tooth-whitening procedures for themselves. This seemed to make sense to Roger, who had recently read in a trade journal that around 500 000 whitening treatments were being carried out each month in the United States and that this figure was growing all the time. Roger left the meeting full of enthusiasm. He felt that his practice was ideally placed to capitalise on this inevitable boom. The next day he ordered a hundred tooth-whitening kits from his local supplier and waited for the flood of new patients to come knocking on his practice door. Nothing much happened for a few weeks. Every now and again Roger managed to persuade one of his patients to have his or her teeth whitened, but it wasn't quite the overwhelming rush he had been hoping for.

Undaunted, he decided to place a series of large adverts in the local newspaper telling people of this wonderful new service his practice was offering. To his surprise and delight, people seemed to be interested in this new development. They had so many questions though: 'Is it dangerous?' 'How long will it last?' and so on. Gill, the girl on the front desk, didn't really know the answers to many of these questions and unbeknown to Roger, who was usually hard at work in the back surgery far away from the reception desk, she could be heard telling callers: 'I know, I agree with you, that is a lot of money and you know we aren't even sure if it's going to work or not!' On occasions during the day Gill was spending so much time on the phone talking about tooth whitening that existing patients began to complain that they couldn't get through to make appointments. Not to worry, Roger thought, they will keep coming back, just as they always had done in the past. Some of the people making enquiries did decide to take the plunge and came in for the whitening procedures. Soon Roger began to wonder if it would not be more cost-effective to employ someone to make the bleaching trays in-house rather than using his usual laboratory – after all, he had to do something to recoup the cost of those adverts. He wasn't too sure where this person would actually be housed, as the practice was already quite cramped. He also realised a decent intra-oral camera would be useful to monitor the whitening process, something he hadn't had much use for in the past.

Six months after the adverts had been placed Roger was beginning to wonder if his love affair with bleach hadn't been a little misguided. Many of the patients who came in for whitening never came back and, even worse, several of his regular patients had defected to his main rival down the road. He was the proud owner of a large carton of unused tooth-whitening kits that were rapidly approaching their sell-by date, and his staff still didn't believe that the procedure worked and offered value for money. If only he had given it a bit more thought . . .

This case demonstrates an almost total absence of a strategic approach involving the following basic steps:
- developing a clear vision of your ideal future ⇒
- assessing your present situation ⇒
- creating a well-thought-out plan ⇒
- implementing your plan: the need to involve staff members ⇒
- measuring the degree of success or failure.

Developing a clear vision of your ideal future

This of course harks back to Strategy 1. Somewhere in Roger Bell's mind was a hazy vision of the future. A future where lots of patients would be coming to see him to have their teeth whitened. Unfortunately, this vision was just too narrow and too blurred. Was this the only change he foresaw for his practice? Did the introduction of a private aesthetic service signal a move away from the NHS towards a more independent style of practice? Did he envisage introducing other related services such as all-porcelain crowns, even making his practice amalgam-free? What impact would all this have on his existing clientele? Knowing where you want to go in the first place, having a clear vision of your 'ideal' future, is an essential first step in strategic planning and will be discussed in greater detail in the next chapter.

Assessing your present situation

This stage in the strategic process requires an objective appraisal of your existing strengths and weaknesses and a need to place these within the context of the prevailing business and professional environment. Roger ran a busy, almost wholly NHS, practice. The strength of this practice was its ability to offer patients a relatively low-cost service comprising basic, conventional dental treatments. The fact that this is what his staff were so used to providing could also be seen as a weakness, in that they might have difficulty in adapting to any fundamental change in practice philosophy. It should have been possible for Roger to anticipate that this problem would arise, but unfortunately he made the mistake of looking only at his practice's strengths and not at its weaknesses as well. An almost total misreading of the wider business and social environment compounded this error. Maybe there are half a million plus whitening treatments being carried out in the United States each month, maybe the visiting lecturer's assessment of an increasing demand was correct . . . in the south-east of England, but did that necessarily translate into the good people of Roger's town joining the throng of masses demanding tooth whitening? A little more market research would have saved Roger a whole lot of trouble later on. Casting a critical eye over your existing strengths and weaknesses, rating the skills of your staff (good, indifferent or poor?) and trying to gauge the prevailing business environment are important elements of any strategic planning process.

Creating a well-thought-out plan

Roger's plan, which really only involved buying the boxes of bleach, was piecemeal in the extreme and simply not sufficiently thought through. Any planning exercise needs a plan, a carefully considered document that converts the leadership's vision into feasible actions that will in turn bring about the hoped-for changes. It is not enough having a great idea of *what* you want to happen; you also need to articulate *how* it is going to be done and *who* is going to do it. It follows, therefore, that any plan must take everyone involved through the various changes, explaining in detail the proposed sequence of events, each individual's level of involvement, what is expected of them, and so on.

Implementing your plan: the need to involve staff members

Strategic analysis is simple, it is implementation that is difficult and it is almost always the human element that complicates the process. It is one of the fundamental principles of strategic planning that any plan will only truly work if it has the backing and involvement of the organisation's workforce. This book's primary theme, one that recurs throughout, is the need to get others to participate. Staff will believe more strongly in a plan if they feel they have contributed to its formulation. An additional reason for involving them is that they often have a better idea of what will work and what won't. As Cyril Levicki[6] writes in his book *Strategy Workout*:

> *The simple answer to the question of who should implement strategy is that everybody should. That is the only way the organization can move cohesively in one direction. It requires wise and sensitive insight into what motivates both large and small groups of people. Persuading them to adapt their behavior to achieve new and different objectives is the highest and most supreme aspect of the art of leadership.*

The attitudes, beliefs and, indeed, behaviour of the people working in an organisation define its culture, a rather abstract set of values that you cannot see or touch but can certainly feel. Even a practice as small as Roger Bell's has a culture, and one of the problems of his approach was that he totally ignored the effect his staff would have on even as small a change as the introduction of tooth-whitening procedures into his practice. He made the mistake of thinking that they would automatically see things the way he did, that they would see the value of the changes being made and that they would pass these new beliefs onto patients. It is impossible to plan strategic changes in any organisation without taking into account its culture and the people who come together to create that culture.

Measuring the degree of success or failure

Roger did make some effort to review his plan, although in the end this amounted to little more than a rather sad admission of defeat. It doesn't appear that he actually learned anything from the whole exercise and would probably repeat the same mistakes once the memory had faded and the next 'big thing' came along. Many strategic planning exercises fail because they do not build in a formal review to assess how well the plan has been implemented and if the original vision has been achieved.

It may well be that in Roger's situation, a move away from an NHS-style of practice would make sense, but such a radical change cannot be carried out lightly and on a whim. Roger needs to sit down and work out exactly where he wants his practice to be in both one year's and three years' time. He needs to make a careful assessment of the response of his staff to such a move and the impact it will have on his patient base. Careful and detailed planning covering every aspect of the change needs to be thought out and written down. In other words, he needs to think *strategically*. We all know how complex dental practice can be, how many variables exist in even the simplest of decisions, how everything can seem to teeter on the edge of chaos when trying to juggle the different needs and demands of patients, staff, laboratories, suppliers, local authorities and regulatory bodies. The primary advantage of thinking strategically is that the strategy itself, the plan of action (however simple or complex) will be all that much better for harnessing the knowledge and ideas of your staff, 'an infinite permutation of moods, abilities and aspirations', who will in turn:

- understand the strategy and be more likely to recognise its importance
- know where their energies should be focused
- appreciate the need to cooperate and work as a team
- not have to try to guess what you want from them
- not require repeated explanations of what you want from them
- be more motivated and energised to work for the good of the practice.

Over 70 years ago, Dr Irvin Tulkin[7] asked the question: '*Can success in dentistry be planned?*' The answer he gave was an unqualified *yes!* In that respect, dentistry hasn't changed all that much.

REFERENCES

1. Shugars DA, DiMatteo MR, Hays RD, *et al*. Professional satisfaction among California general dentists. *J Dent Educ*. 1990; **54**(11): 661–9.
2. Cooper CL, Watts J, Kelly M. Job satisfaction, mental health, and job stressors among general dental practitioners in the UK. *Br Dent J*. 1987; **162**(2): 77–81.
3. www.strategiccoach.com
4. Beckwith H. *Selling the Invisible: A field guide to modern marketing*. New York: Warner Books; 2012.
5. Solomon M, Bamossy G, Askegaard S *et al*. *Consumer Behaviour: A European perspective*. 4th ed. London Prentice Hall; 2010.

6. Levicki C. *Strategy Workout: Analyze and develop the fitness of your business.* 2nd ed. London: Prentice Hall; 2003.
7. Tulkin I. Can success in dentistry be planned? *Dental Items of Interest.* 1942; **64**: 134–44.

CHAPTER FOUR

Strategy 3: Control your finances

Money is a good servant but a bad master.

Francis Bacon

It is a fact that after three to four years, 90 out of 100 new businesses have failed. Bank managers will tell you that the reason is because they don't manage their finances correctly. After 10 years, only one out of 100 new businesses will remain. Why? Lack of financial control.

Short of illness, there aren't many things worse than financial stress. It really is one of the most miserable places to be – sleepless nights, an inability to focus on the job at hand and the gradual deterioration of one's passion for a chosen vocation. From our own experience we estimate that around 20% of dentists are in some form of financial trouble. Perhaps we should not be too surprised by this because, despite the fact that money and dentistry have gone together since time immemorial, business and financial matters are seldom taught at dental school. This is primarily because the people who teach in these institutions have little grasp of such things themselves. Most dental academics fit the description of 'poor dad' – salaried, non-entrepreneurial and risk-averse – in one of our favourite books, *Rich Dad, Poor Dad* by Robert Kiyosaki and Sharon Lechter.[1] This is one of those books you wish you had read 25 years ago – it is a simple but profoundly effective guide to making money work for you instead of you working for money.

If you are thinking, *'well, I'm alright'*, we need to warn you that it's dangerous to be complacent, especially in a marketplace that is evolving as rapidly as dentistry. All those changes we described in Chapter One have created a competitive melting pot in which you must keep your eye on the commercial ball if you intend to survive and prosper over the next 10 years. So let's take a look at money and what we believe to be the seven top tactics (*see* Box 4.1) you can employ to ensure that:

- in the short-term your business comfortably generates your desired standard of living and pays its bills
- in the medium-term, your finances are becoming more attractive each year
- ultimately, in the long-term, you are building 'financial independence' – whatever that means to you. This does not necessarily mean building the biggest pile of money; more, being able to do what you want to do, with whom you want and when you want.

BOX 4.1 Seven steps for maintaining financial control

1. Create budgets (on a personal and professional basis)
2. Create monthly management accounts
3. Look at your financial results
4. Make course corrections
5. Get your prices right
6. Reduce debt
7. Build reserves

The benefits of incorporating these new habits are:
- increased sense of control
- increased self-control and self-esteem
- significant drop in stress levels.

WHAT IS *YOUR* DEFINITION OF SUCCESS?

This may not necessarily be in terms of how much money you make. For many people 'success' is doing what you want to do – with people you want to do it with – when you want to do it. Take a few minutes to consider your own definition of success and write your thoughts down.

 My definition of success is:

STEP 1: PREPARE PERSONAL AND PROFESSIONAL BUDGETS

We begin by encouraging you to take the time off around each October to prepare projected expenditure budgets, both personally and professionally, for the following calendar year. This should be an uninterrupted couple of days and preferably somewhere away from work. If possible, use a spreadsheet program, such as Microsoft Excel, to list all personal expenses, including luxury items, for the next 12 months. For your professional budget, detail fixed costs, overheads and any projected capital expenditure.

When CB worked as an independent financial advisor, he used to tell the following story:

> *Imagine that the government has introduced a new system for collecting money from businesses. You are allowed to keep all the cash patients pay you for the complete calendar year and you don't have to pay any bills whatsoever.*
>
> *On New Year's Eve a giant cash till is constructed outside your dental practice and your creditors line up to take their share. Who is first in the queue?*

The answer is Her Majesty's Revenue and Customs followed by your staff for their wages if the business is solvent and statutory redundancy pay if the business is bust. Next in the queue will be your secured creditors (those to whom you've given a charge on bricks and mortar), next come unsecured creditors (mainly your trade creditors) and – finally – at the stroke of midnight you, the principal, the owner of the business, the person who took the risk, the one who lies awake at night worrying about everything. You can take whatever is left in the till home. By preparing your personal expenditure budget one year in advance, you are putting yourself at the front of the queue. The total income you require for the year becomes the first line in the budget that you prepare for your potential business expenditure.

Imagine that your total personal expenses for the year are budgeted to be £60 000 before the payment of any tax. That includes your necessities, your optional expenses and the luxuries that you build in, such as holidays, clothing, entertainment, and so on. You may then arbitrarily apply a factor of say 30% for taxation and gross this up to around £90 000, pre-tax. This then is the first line on your professional budget to which you would add the fixed cost, overheads and capital costs that we already mentioned. So, let's say that the overall gross revenue target for the year is £200 000.

We'll talk about pricing later, but for the moment let's accept that in business, once you have calculated your gross revenue target for the year, you only have three potential ways of breaking that target down during the year itself.

1. Divide the gross by the amount of time available; for example, I plan to work

200 clinical days next year so my gross revenue target is £1000 a day. I plan to work 8 hours clinical each day so my hourly rate is approximately £120; therefore, every price I quote to patients is made of 'average time', plus lab fees.

2. Divide the gross by the number of clients who you intend to deal with (very difficult to achieve in dentistry).

3. Divide the gross revenues by the unit price of sales. As far as we can see, the only group in dentistry that could do this would be specialists; for example, an endodontist could argue that to achieve a gross revenue target of £200 000 while working 100 clinical days with eight appointments a day. The rate would, therefore, be £250 (200 000/(100 × 8)) per patient.

For dentists in general practice, their prices will most often be expressed as average time, plus lab fees. Budgets establish the prices. Once the year begins, it is necessary to compare budgets versus actual expenditure on a monthly basis and make appropriate adjustments to the overall gross revenue target for the year and, subsequently, to the prices that you charge. For this reason, we advocate a revised price list every three months.

If you need new equipment, to recruit an extra member of staff, or to refurbish the surgery, then there are only two groups of people who can pay – either you (and your family) or the patient. You can't gather your staff together and say, *'I've just bought a new car so I'd like you all to take a 5% pay cut.'* Therefore, any increase in costs *must* be passed on as an increase in prices.

It's your choice – would you rather work like crazy for 364 days and then look in the till at the end of the year to see what's left or decide, in advance, what you want your pre-tax income to be and then spend the next 364 days making it happen?

STEP 2: PREPARE MONTHLY MANAGEMENT ACCOUNTS

The budgets that we have just talked about are the number-one tactic for you to run your businesses and financial lives – the old cliché 'cash is king' is undoubtedly true. An extremely tight control of cash flow and projected cash flow is necessary to ensure your financial well-being. However, we still need to produce accounts because they are a means by which:

• the Inland Revenue can keep score and charge us tax
• banks and other lenders can assess our credit-worthiness
• we can measure trends in our business to determine whether there are any subtle increases in our costs, which need to be passed on to the customer.

Monthly accounts ensure you express every category of expenditure as a percentage of gross revenues for that month. The figures are not important, but the percentages are. For example, if we see that your lab costs move from 12% to 12.5% and then up to 13% of gross revenues over a three-month period, that could be telling us:

- the lab put their fees up
- you have started to use higher-quality materials
- perhaps you are seeing more private patients
- there is some factor we need to identify that is affecting these costs.

Your accounts should look at everything – staff costs, lab fees, utility bills, other materials and dental supplies, petrol, everything – so that you can determine what's happening. If there has been an increase in your costs, then you must choose to either reduce your standard of living or pass the increases onto your customers. One last thing: if at all possible, delegate this function to a bookkeeper. It will save you many hours of work, which you can use far more profitably doing other things.

STEP 3: LOOK AT YOUR FINANCIAL RESULTS

How often do you call a meeting, away from work, free from interruptions, mobile phones switched off, in which to monitor your financial progress and make plans for the future? In Strategy 2 we looked at free, focus and buffer days. Remember buffer days = business development days = days on which you consider financial results. It is imperative to schedule time each month to evaluate your financial results, review management accounts, compare them with your budgets and then make course corrections as needed. Make it an agenda item at the monthly board meeting that we recommended in Strategy 2.

To recap, the board meeting should include a five-point agenda: (1) finance, (2) sales, (3) marketing, (4) resources and (5) personnel. When discussing finance, you might like to:

- review management accounts for the last month
- review management accounts for the last year to date
- compare management accounts with budget
- make required course corrections
- assess the current cash flow situation
- decide what action needs to be taken to accelerate cash flow
- review the current pricing strategy.

Who should be present?

- *If your business is a one-man band*: make an appointment with yourself to do this.
- *Small business*: yourself and the practice manager.
- *Larger business*: yourself and all partners, directors, and external consultants, such as your accountant and banker, although they may only need to come in occasionally.

What should I do now?

If you have not already scheduled all your board meetings a year in advance then it is highly recommended that you do so *now*.

Create your own personal board of directors. This is made up of those people you know and trust who can keep you on track. Who do you know who would be willing to be part of your continued success?

STEP 4: MAKE COURSE CORRECTIONS

Running a business is like sailing a yacht. A yacht is susceptible to both external and internal influences – externally, the wind and the tide; internally, the set of the sail and the trim of the boat. Likewise, your business yacht is subject to both external and internal influences: externally, market conditions, taxation, raw material prices; internally, the changes in your desired lifestyle and in your cost of running the business.

Let's imagine that two yachts begin a transatlantic race. They are crewed by people of exactly the same competence who sail for exactly the same number of hours. The first crew sail around the clock as hard as they possibly can, but never navigate, take a positional reading or tack. The second crew sail around the clock, but every hour take a positional reading and tack. Both will expend the same amount of energy, but we have no idea where the first crew will end up. Which of these vessels looks most like your business?

By producing your budgets you have already started plotting a course and a destination. Your monthly meetings are the framework you will use to change course, as dictated by any changes in your financial position, otherwise you will be just as exhausted at the end of the year, but you could arrive anywhere, including troubled waters. Remember:

Consider – Decide – Act.

What needs to happen to get the vessel back on course, or to change direction completely?

- Look at the current cash flow situation: consider how to accelerate cash flow into the business.
- Review your current pricing strategy to reflect increasing costs of business.

More control = Less stress = More confidence!

STEP 5: GET YOUR PRICES RIGHT

We are going to spend some time looking at this last tactic for gaining financial control because it causes so many problems for so many dentists. Let's go all theoretical for a moment and ask the following question . . .

Why is putting a price on dentistry different?

If you were asked to estimate the price of, on the one hand, a CD or, on the other, a service for your car, you would probably be able to provide an answer for both on the basis of memory – the so-called 'internal reference price', which can consist of, for example, the last price paid, or the price most frequently paid. However, with these two items, the CD or the service, which of your estimates do you feel most confident will be closest to the actual price? If you are like most people you will feel quite uncertain about your knowledge of the prices of services, and the reference prices you hold for them in your memory will probably not be as accurate as those you hold for goods (the CD). There are a number of reasons for this difference.

Intangibility

Because services are intangible and are not created on a factory assembly line, service providers have great flexibility and can conceivably offer an infinite variety of pricing combinations and permutations. Life insurance is a prime example, with a multitude of types and variations on offer. Only an expert customer, one who knows enough about the insurance industry to completely specify the options across providers, is likely to find prices that are directly comparable. The same applies to dentistry. So much of the care we provide is intangible in nature – when we provide immediate dentures, for example, we are not just providing an off-the-shelf product but a custom-made item, the success of which is determined not only by the physical characteristics of the dentures themselves but also by our own, very intangible, ability to explain, motivate and encourage. Dental marketing expert Sheila Scott[*] has said that for patients, buying dentistry is like buying a pair of shoes in a black plas-

---

[*] Sheila Scott. Personal communication.

tic bag. You can't see it, touch it or even know if you want or need it in the first place.

Lack of information

Another reason customers lack accurate reference prices for services is that many providers are unable or unwilling to estimate price in advance. The fundamental reason in many cases is that the providers themselves do not know what will be involved until the process of service delivery unfolds, as, for example, in the case of a court trial. Similarly, a dentist can quote for the cost of a crown, but what happens if it is found during preparation that the tooth needs to be root-treated? Does the dentist pass on the cost to the patient who may now feel aggrieved at having to pay more than originally thought, or should he or she do what is described in the United States as 'eating the fee'? One could of course argue that the case should have been better planned or that the dentist should have managed the patient's expectations better by warning of the possibility of a need for root canal therapy. Realistically though, it is difficult to warn patients of every possible complication, however much the dental insurance providers would like us to.

Different patient needs

Another factor that results in the inaccuracy of reference prices is that the needs of individuals vary. If you were to ask a friend the cost of a haircut from a particular stylist the chances are that your cut from the same stylist would be a different price. The same applies to dental care, only more so. Without a good explanation, patients might find it difficult to understand why, for example, their orthodontic treatment costs more than that of their friend's – to most patients braces are braces.

Finally, yet another reason why customers lack accurate reference prices for services is that they feel overwhelmed with the information they need to gather. With most goods, retail stores display the products by categories to allow customers to compare and contrast the prices of different brands. With the growth of the shopping mall this process has become even easier. Rarely is there a similar display of services in a single outlet. If customers want to compare the prices charged by various dentists, they must contact individual practices in person or by phone and even then they may not receive the information they feel that they need.

Price as an indicator of quality

One of the interesting aspects of pricing is that consumers use price as an indicator of the quality of the service and not just its cost, or, put another way,

'Price is at once an attraction and a repellent'. The use of price as an indicator of quality depends on several factors, one of which is the extent to which other information is available to the buyer. When other pointers to quality are readily accessible (the ability to touch and feel the quality of a Chanel suit), when brand names provide evidence of a company's reputation (the Virgin Group is a classic example), or when advertising successfully communicates the company's belief in the brand (take the Volkswagen Group), then customers may prefer to use those pointers instead of price. In other situations, however, such as when quality is hard to detect or when quality or price varies a great deal within a class of services (such as dentistry), consumers may believe that price is the best indicator of quality. A further factor that increases the dependence on price as a quality indicator is the risk associated with the purchase. In high-risk situations, and to most patients complicated dental treatment most certainly falls into this category, people will look to price as a surrogate for quality.

Because patients do often rely on price as a cue to quality and because price does establish certain expectations of quality, the prices set must be determined carefully. So, as well as being chosen to cover costs or match competitors, prices must be chosen to convey the appropriate quality signal. While pricing too high can set expectations that may be difficult to match, pricing too low can lead to inaccurate inferences about the quality of the care provided. This is why competing on price alone is a very risky strategy. It is difficult to imagine a dental practice whose vision centres on the principle of lowest cost, devoting the time and resources to implementing excellent service quality that will ultimately determine whether a person stays loyal to the practice. Price wars may have a brief effect in some industries but dentistry is not one of them, and the public do not like to think they are buying low quality – ask Gerald Ratner, who effectively brought down his family's jewellery business when he described their products as 'crap'.[2] Interestingly, though, Ratner's has reinvented itself as an online business, with its name still the most recognised jewellery brand in the UK! Maybe for all the wrong reasons, but memorable nonetheless. It has been said that bad publicity is like bad breath – it's better than none at all! If you have gone through the steps outlined in the earlier sequence of tactics it is likely that your conclusion will be that you have to raise prices.

> CB: *Our clients on average increase their prices by around 30% in the first 12 months of business coaching without any significantly adverse reaction from patients. So it would seem that general dentistry has not yet reached anything remotely like its emotional price-resistance level in the market place.*

The idea of raising fees is quite emotive for most dentists. It sounds so logical but the suggestion is usually met with 'patients will leave in droves'. If, however, you offer a five-star service, where are they going to go? To that dentist down the road who is cheaper but offers a much inferior patient experience? Have confidence in the prices you charge but, and it's a big but, make sure you offer that five-star service and patients will not leave in droves. One study that appeared in the *British Dental Journal* some years ago showed that 19% of people said their reason for changing dentist was because the dentist was 'too expensive' and a further 6% said it was because the dentist had 'gone private'.[3] However, the remaining 75% gave a whole collection of reasons unrelated to price – for example, 'unhappy with dentist' (26%); 'retired/closed/died' (16%); 'unhappy with work' (8%); 'poor appointments/rushed' (4%); 'recommended to better practice' (3%); 'rough dentist/painful' (3%); 'closer/more convenient' (3%); 'rude/bad tempered' (2%). Price, then, is unquestionably a factor but not the major one in deciding whether a patient stays with you or jumps ship to another practice.

Going rate pricing

Picking up on the theme developed earlier, we believe that general dental practice prices should always be based on 'average time'. It also worth saying now that with very few exceptions we feel strongly that there are no such things as loss leaders – loss leaders are loss makers. The situation often arises where the dentist decides to sell the initial examination or routine check-up at a rate much lower than the hourly rate required to maintain practice viability. Unfortunately, when the time comes to sell any treatment (if ever), the dentist often forgets to charge an enhanced hourly rate. You must be very clear therefore about:

- what your rates are for different treatments
- what skills you have in the practice to expose yourself to the risks of doing business!

One criticism of this pricing approach is that it tends to ignore demand factors and competitors' prices. The price charged by competitors for similar or substitute services may determine where, within the ceiling-to-floor range, the price level should actually be pitched. The more information one can gather about the fees charged by your competitors and the reactions of people to those prices, the easier it will be to establish where prices might be set. Such 'going-rate pricing' is quite popular in professional services. However, since it is based largely on competitors' prices, with less attention being paid to cost or demand, it can be seen that copycat pricing usually fails to set the optimal price.

Perceived value pricing

The approaches to pricing dental care described so far are based on (a) the dental practice and (b) its competitors rather than on patients. A third approach to pricing therefore involves setting prices consistent with patient perceptions of value: prices are based on what patients will pay for the services provided. Demand is the result of the consumer's perception of value. The nature of any transaction, whatever the product – tangible good or intangible service – is such that customers make judgements about what they get in return for what they give. The concept of *differential advantage* holds that the best-performing organisations are those that offer the greatest customer value and are able to sustain that value over time.[4]

Perceived-value pricing sees the buyer's perception of value, not the seller's cost, as the key to pricing. It allows for the use of non-price variables in the marketing mix to build up perceived value in the buyer's mind. Price is then set to capture the perceived value. Perceived-value pricing fits well with modern marketing thinking, which sees products or services being developed for particular target markets with planned quality and price. The key to perceived-value pricing is to accurately determine the market's perception of the offer's value. Sellers with an inflated view of the value of their offer will overprice the product. Alternatively, they may underestimate the perceived value and charge less than they could. Clearly, market research is needed to establish the market's perception of value as a guide to effective pricing.

To understand this in terms of dental practice one must consider what exactly is being sold – are you selling the crown itself or the benefits that accrue from that crown? Salisbury dentist Charles Lister[*] puts it this way:

> *We are selling our professional services, not items of treatment. The patients pay our fees for the benefits they receive in return – good dental health, dental wellbeing, comfort, nicer smiles and not the mechanics of how this is achieved. We therefore need to set our rates accordingly, to allow us to live comfortably, have enough free time, time for planning and administration, and to show a profit that allows re-investment for the long-term benefit of our practices and our patients.*

Communicating the fee to the patient

Whichever approach is chosen, the dentist is still confronted by the dilemma of choosing the most appropriate way and time to communicate the prices to the patient. If you have followed our arguments so far you will see why, along with a growing number of dentists, we believe that prices for individual items

---

[*] Lister C. Personal communication; 2002.

of treatment should not be shown to patients, even if they are the basis upon which the fees have been set. Instead, the patient is quoted a global sum, with the actual price list merely used as a reference by the dentist. Well-known private practitioner Barry Posner* says:

> Don't hand out prices to all and sundry. How many patients will understand anything more than a very simple description which will fall short of describing and valuing a very high-tech procedure.

What is especially clear is that patients do prefer to know the cost implications as early on as possible and do not appreciate going through a course of treatment oblivious of the bill that will be facing them at the end of treatment.[5] It has been suggested that dentists have difficulty with both set-fee scales and hourly rates because they have not convinced themselves that their fees offer value for money for high-quality dental care. Barry Posner[†] again:

> Ever been faced on the phone with a query and swallowing hard before you force out the words 'two thousand pounds'? Fear of rejection? Don't say it, read it. It is very much easier. Don't say 'about . . .', to soften the blow. Don't ever say 'I'm sorry but . . .'. Harrods don't label carpets in their window with 'We're sorry but these carpets are about five thousand pounds each.' All this stems from Colin Hall Dexter's 'neuro-fiscal drag'. Your brain thinks one thousand and your voice says five hundred.

Our take on this is that if you advertise your hourly rate as £160, you may well receive lots of negative feedback from individuals who'll tell you that they only pay their accountant £100 per hour and their solicitor £90 per hour, so why should they pay you £160? Unwittingly, one of the greatest business coaches in the world may have been the late Irish comedian Frank Carson who coined the phrase 'It's the way I tell 'em'. It is not necessary for you to quote your hourly rate. It is necessary for you to quote an accurate price and to back that up with a detailed and transparent treatment plan.

If you intend to allocate 30 minutes to a routine examination and your hourly rate is £160, then a routine examination costs £80. If you intend to spend two hours on a crown over two appointments then the price of a crown is £320, plus the lab fee, and so it goes on. The problem with this is that dentists feel they can't charge £80 for a routine examination – and we can understand

---

* Postner B. Personal communication; 2002.
† Ibid.

that. It's for that reason that the private patient member scheme is such a wonderful business model.

By way of example, the absolute bottom line for patients is to attend the practice for two examinations a year (each of 30 minutes' duration) and two visits to the hygienist (each of 20 minutes' duration). Now we know that our dentist is charging £160 per hour, so the two examinations cost £160. Let's assume that we are charging the hygienist's time at £60 per hour, so the two hygiene visits are going to cost £40. This means annual cost of basic dental maintenance is £200. Your private membership scheme therefore costs £200, which you can divide over 12 monthly direct debit payments and include administration charges and perhaps a nominal monthly charge for emergency insurance. Consequently, in this case, the type of clients that you want to attract are those who are going to be happy to pay around £18 per month for the maintenance of their dental health.

Of course, most of the external providers of membership schemes services will also suggest that you offer patients some form of discount on the fee-per-item price list as a reward for joining the basic membership scheme. This business model seems so crushingly logical that we sometimes find it difficult to understand how anybody would want to communicate their prices any other way.

Collection policy

Setting fees may in fact be the easiest part. Where most dentists come unstuck is in their failure to define and then implement a strict collection policy. Collection is a huge issue in dental practice and one that is paid only scant attention. American practice management guru Dr Rick Kushner[6] says that collection policy is one of the cornerstones of successful practice, noting that most practices have a *billing* policy but not a *collection* policy. In relatively complex cases, for example, he advocates offering patients a number of alternatives such as a cash discount for full payment upfront or a pay-as-you-go option with payment due on each day any particular component of the treatment plan is provided, *before* the patient enters the surgery. Most people feel that a full payment – made pre-treatment and perhaps with a discount – is the most favourable option (despite the aforementioned problem of how to deal with unforeseen treatment needs) in that it eliminates the risk of bad debts and makes patient attendance and compliance more likely. Kushner warns that the pay-as-you-go is more fraught with problems – primarily, the situation that can arise where the patient attends but doesn't bring any money: '*I forgot my cheque book.*' The temptation is to go ahead and carry out the treatment and then bill the patient for the money owed. This, says, Kushner is a fundamental error made by many dentists. He advocates that dentists inform the patient that the work cannot be done that day and recommends them to reschedule the appointment. Kushner's argument is that most dentists do too much work effectively for free and end up with poor collection rates and ensuing bad debts, something he terms 'overproduction'.

> *I am a big supporter of positive internal marketing or patient relations, yet I have this hard-nosed collection policy. Not so. It is a firm, but fair, policy, and we know that the hard feelings develop when dentistry is done and then we 'hound' payment. When it is all tied up neat and tidy, the patient relations remain strong. You know what else? Patients like the dentistry much better when it's paid for. Go through your account cards or your software and identify which patients are not active . . . those who owe money![6]*

This is clearly quite a controversial approach, one that has made Rick Kushner a rather notorious figure in the United States, but nevertheless one that at least deserves to be listened to.

The following are some tips on what to do with bad payers.
- Be sure to include payment terms in your business literature.
- Repeat your payment terms in any treatment plans.
- Remind clients to bring payment means with them prior to a fee-paying appointment.
- Have automated payment facilities on-site (credit cards).
- If they fail to make a payment on the spot, send the invoice with a self-addressed envelope. Include on the invoice a paragraph to say that your normal terms are 30 days and that in excess of 30 days there will be an administration fee payable and also add the phrase 'Please help small businesses by paying promptly'.

And what to do about broken appointments:
- Spell out your terms and conditions clearly in your business literature – then people don't have the right to complain.
- Many practices tell patients that if they cancel with more than 24 hours notice then there will be no charge. We ask what is so special about 24 hours – it is still disruptive – and so now an increasing number of practices request credit card confirmation of all appointment bookings and suggest that a cancellation fee will always be charged unless there is a 'genuine' emergency, when discretion will be used. This will catch persistent offenders.
- Within 24 hours you are granted one free missed appointment per year. Every time after that you pay the cost of each missed appointment.

STEP 6: REDUCE DEBT

In our experience there are two types of debt:

1. *Normal debt* = investment or business debt = non-speculative debt, secured against assets (property) the objective of which is to put money to work – medium- and long-term debt.
2. *Stupid debt* = consumer debt = any debt designed to finance the purchase of a consumable, not secured against assets (e.g. credit card, bank loans, overdraft, asset finance – short-term debt, on which we are usually paying a ridiculously high rate of interest). Current statistics for the UK population as a whole make depressing reading – money owed on credit cards is £21 billion, while money owed on overdrafts stands at around £6 billion.

Let's face it, most of us sometimes run up a stupid debt; perhaps when we have used a credit or debit card to finance an expenditure that wasn't budgeted for, but we have had a rush of blood and want to reward ourselves either professionally or personally. Most of us know, though, how much it hurts when we open that credit card statement and they tell us that they have charged another 19% interest.

As far as debt is concerned, you should have two objectives:

1. to reduce or eliminate the extent to which you get involved in stupid debt
2. to have a plan to eliminate normal debt completely from your life as rapidly as possible, with the exception of leveraged property investment.

If you are budgeting properly, debt reduction simply becomes an additional line in your personal and professional expenditure cash flows. This should mean that it's the patients who pay off your debt, not you.

Sometimes it is necessary for us to put some safeguards in place to prevent getting into debt because of those rushes of blood that we mentioned earlier. It is understandable that if the business is doing well and cash flow is healthy, you might have an overwhelming urge to go out and buy yourself some new toys, either personally or professionally. Once you have the business in shape, you can then create some extra lines in your budgets for the year, which relate to 'accelerated debt repayment'. For instance, if you have a domestic mortgage that is due to be repaid in 15 years' time, work out how much extra you would have to pay now in order to clear the mortgage in 10 years. Add that to the lines in your budgets, adjust your prices and see what difference it makes. For example, if by increasing your prices by 2% you could reduce your mortgage repayments from 15 years to 10 years, would you be interested? Would the patients notice?

STEP 7: BUILD RESERVES

How would it feel to have *much* more than enough money, energy, time, love, space, support, skill and nourishing relationships?

One of the characteristics of successful people is that they have reserves. Reserves are massively important in life, and the number-one reason for this is because the existence of reserves gives us the ability to say 'no' to people and to personal and business opportunities that we do not wish to take part in. You no longer make decisions based on 'need'. In terms of finances, why just have 'enough'? Develop an *abundance* mentality. When you go for it – guess what – it happens!

Write down your profit target for this year: £_____

Is there any reason why you shouldn't double it? What steps would you need to take to achieve this?

Having reserves means that you don't have to tolerate patients who mess you about. Having reserves means that you don't need to tolerate staff members who are taking you for a ride. Having reserves means that you can negotiate with suppliers to get the best possible price and enhance your profitability. Having reserves means that you tell the bank what you want from them. Having reserves means that you can cope with the emergencies that will occur.

Although the context of this section of the book is the control of finances, we feel obliged to point out that it is not just about money. It's important to have reserves of money, time, energy, talent, love, space, and so on. As far as financial reserves are concerned, build into your budgets a provision that will have allowed you to completely eliminate all stupid debts from your life within three years. Perhaps within 10 years you will have eliminated all normal debt other than that which you are using for property investment purposes.

REFERENCES

1. Kiyosaki R, Lechter S. *Rich Dad, Poor Dad.* Warner Books; 2011.
2. Doing a Ratner' and other famous gaffes. *The Daily Telegraph* (London). 22 December 2007.
3. Holt VP, McHugh K. Factors influencing patient loyalty to dentist and dental practice. *Br Dent J.* 1997; **183**(10): 365–70.

4. Porter M. *Competitive Strategy: Techniques for analyzing industries and competitors.* New York, NY: Free Press; 2004.
5. Newsome PR, Wright GH. Qualitative techniques to investigate how patients evaluate dentists: a pilot study. *Community Dent Oral Epidemiol.* 2000; **28**(4): 257–66.
6. Kushner R. Collection policy for the next millennium. *Simple Truth.* 1997; **2**: 8–13.

CHAPTER FIVE

Strategy 4: Lead a championship support team

If you look for the best in your employees, they'll flourish. If you criticise or look for the worst, they'll shrivel up. We all need lots of watering.

Richard Branson

The irresistible practice can only become irresistible when it is staffed and run by an irresistible team of people. We would go as far as to say that we have never seen a truly successful practice without the presence of such a team. This is not to say that the staff in other practices are not special human beings – everyone is special – more that they do not gel and function (or are not given the opportunity to do so) and do not possess that certain something that grabs the attention of others. Robert Hamric[1] said as much when he observed: 'You will never see a million-dollar practice without a million-dollar staff' and came to the conclusion that the top four factors for success in dental practice were staff that are:

1. exceptional
2. well paid
3. likeable and people-oriented
4. highly trained in customer service.

People who come to your practice are placing their trust in you and one of the key tasks for you and your team is to nurture that trust and to strengthen the confidence people have in you and in what you stand for. There must be *no doubt at all* in their minds that they have come to the right place for their dental treatment and that they feel just so fortunate to have sought out and found such a fabulous caring practice amid the rough seas of dental uncertainty and mediocrity.

Clearly you cannot do this entirely on your own; you need the total support and backing of your team to turn your dreams into reality. This goes back to the ideas discussed in Strategy 1 of creating a vision and sharing that with the group of people you surround yourself with. Selecting the right people to work with you is critical. A favourite phrase of ours is 'Attitude not aptitude determines altitude', or, as an editorial in the *Journal of the American Dental Association* put it, 'Hire for attitude, train for skill'.[2] In other words, people can be trained to fulfil the technical aspects of a particular job but it is almost impossible to change a person's underlying character. You can train most people to handle a practice software system but it is much more difficult to train someone to smile warmly and genuinely if it is just not in their nature to do so. That said, even the most cheery, personable of people will lose heart if their working conditions are poor.

What little research that has been done in the area of staff management in dental practice suggests that staff – in particular, dental surgery assistants (DSAs) – are often unhappy with their work. There are an estimated 27 000 DSAs in the UK. They have a short working life – four to five years on average – which suggests that they are not all that happy with their jobs. One study carried out in Canada by behavioural expert David Locker and colleagues[3] showed job stress to be common and often severe among DSAs. The same has been found in the UK, with considerably higher levels of stress and dissatisfaction among DSAs than with other dental staff. More and more qualitative research is being done in this area and this tends to shed greater light on the cause and nature of this stress and the ensuing job dissatisfaction. For example, one study conducted by Blinkhorn[4] and based on discussions among groups of DSAs from general practice highlighted two major sources of stress. First, DSAs characterised the managerial style of many dentists as 'self-centred' and overcritical of other staff. The dentists tended to assume that DSAs would stay late (often unpaid) to cover overrunning clinics. The DSA would, as a result, feel treated as a 'non-person'. Second, general working conditions were mentioned: low status and salary and long working hours. Sounds far removed from the sort of environment that would cultivate Robert Hamric's[1] 'Million-dollar staff', doesn't it?

Another study, conducted in the Community Dental Service of North Wales, showed that DSAs feel their work is highly controlled by others.[5] Perceived control has been shown to be a good predictor of job satisfaction, and the study suggested strategies that might improve a sense of perceived control, including:
- enhancing the involvement of staff in the practice management process
- greater consultation with staff

- clarity over what is expected of them
- regular reviews and negotiation over the rewards for the job.

A follow-up to Blinkhorn's[4] study confirmed that regular staff meetings, annual salary reviews and clear job descriptions were indeed associated with significantly less job stress.[6] However, only 19% of the DSAs surveyed worked in practices that held regular staff meetings, although over 60% did have regular salary reviews and clear job descriptions. It seems reasonable to assume that the dentists running those practices where these management measures were commonplace also tended to foster good relations in general.

Finally, let's look at one fascinating study by Maria Mindak[7] comparing the views of DSAs *and* dentists on the role played by DSAs in 20 dental practices in the South Thames region. The majority of dentists felt that the nurse's role should be to anticipate their needs, while the nurses were more concerned about putting the needs of the patient first. Nurses also felt that their role was stressful (surprise, surprise) and reported a lack of praise and recognition of their efforts by dentists (ditto). Few practices had written contracts or performance appraisals. Conclusion . . . a lack of effective communication in many dental practices, producing role strain for the nurse and reduced job satisfaction.

All of these studies are telling us that DSAs want their efforts recognised and acknowledged by the dentist yet they feel that this rarely occurs – remember the old adage about *praise*, the gift we all yearn to receive but find so difficult to give. When recognition does occur, it is much appreciated and contributes to a better working environment in the practice, which is then noticed by patients. The following two widely contrasting quotes taken from two different DSAs interviewed in Maria Mindak's study encapsulate all of this:

> *He just expected everything there without telling you or asking you. Me sitting there not doing it because I don't know what he needs and him probably thinking, 'Oh she's just sitting there', but it's not, it's because he's not actually explained what he needs and therefore I can't mix it when I don't know.*

> *I think really a dentist should include their nurse in their work or they can make them feel just like the washer-upper and I feel very included here . . . he's terrific, absolutely terrific. This dentist will at the end of the day say 'thank you'. That's not usual, normally they're tools down and gone and leave you to clear up.*[7]

These research findings are telling you what is happening in hundreds of practices up and down the country, in your competitors' practices and, quite possibly if you are honest with yourself, even in your own practice. Can you honestly say that your team exhibits all the signs that Paddi Lund[8] has said defines the 'happy practice':

- people stay a long time with your business – long-term team, customers and suppliers
- people smile and laugh a lot
- people do not complain constantly about their conditions, money, hours, standard of service, wages, bills, and so forth
- people come early and leave late; they like to spend time at your place of business
- people talk with one another in a friendly way
- people are polite to one another
- people do not gossip and backbite
- when you ask people about one another, their comments are complimentary.

This is not to say that everyone should agree over everything all the time. There are times when someone has to say if a problem exists and, indeed, Tim Kemp[9] says you should ask yourself whether your practice is an environment where:

- differences are valued
- alternative views are expected and sought
- people feel able to disagree
- different people take responsibility for challenging established routines or procedures
- conflict is seen as healthy
- disagreements are explored, not smoothed over
- everybody is able to identify areas of disagreement
- people feel able to 'agree to disagree'
- old unfinished arguments do not reappear.

These two lists are not mutually exclusive but what is critically important is that any disagreements are aired in private and not in front of patients. The need for an appropriate forum for discussion is vital. Taking these ideas a little further, consider the all-too-common sequence of events represented in Figure 5.1.

If we start off in the lower right-hand box we find our new recruit, often with little in the way of technical skills but brimming with enthusiasm. We can describe this person as 'ignorance on fire' – can't wait to learn about the job, eager to help, desperate to climb up the career ladder. If we are lucky, this person will soon move up to the top right-hand box. With correct training and lots and lots of encouragement our new recruit gains technical skills while at

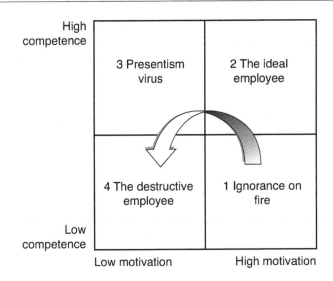

FIGURE 5.1 Motivation and competence – two parameters that help us assess our employees

the same time maintaining that oh-so-appealing enthusiasm. This is also the box in which we want all our team members to stay. Of course there is probably no end to the amount of training that can be done to hone and polish technical skills, but the difficulty lies in maintaining enthusiasm. The problem is that enthusiasm tends to wane unless the person is, to quote Richard Branson, 'watered'. Without due care and attention it is so easy for a skilful, valued employee to slip across into the top left-hand box. We use the word 'presentism' to describe these employees – they turn up for work, do the job, but their hearts and minds are somewhere else. Such people possess all the requisite skills but are lacking motivation and enthusiasm for the work they do. Given the previously quoted statistic of the average working life of a DSA being around five years, then for many employees this phase probably happens as early as the third or fourth year. The longer the time people spend in this box the more likely they are to 'infect' others with their negative attitude, hence the use of the word virus. Better to try to avoid anyone reaching this stage, because getting them back to the top right-hand box can be difficult indeed, and it is almost inevitable that they will sooner rather than later slip down into the mire that is the bottom left-hand box. Here, motivation is shot to pieces and as a result there is no incentive to maintain technical skills – end result, an employee who will either leave of his or her own accord or one who will eventually be asked to leave.

So, what strategies and tactics can you adopt in order to build a winning, motivated team where every member of that team, including yourself, is nestled safely in the top right-hand box . . . or at least is heading towards it from the direction of the bottom right-hand one? Read on.

As you will know by now, one of our core philosophies is that you should spend 80% of your time pursuing your unique ability and 20% leading the support staff who have the responsibility for carrying out everything else in the practice. Notice the presence of the word 'leading' in this philosophy?

LEADERSHIP

Leadership is one of the most talked about and one of the least understood phenomena in management these days, with hundreds of definitions of what it takes to be an effective leader. It is clear that autocratic ways relying on fear and intimidation are slowly being consigned to the dustbin, to be replaced by leadership through communication and guidance. It is important to realise from the outset that leading people and managing them are not one and the same thing and that we should try to distinguish between the two concepts – even if, in most small organisations (including dental practices), the same person assumes the two roles. Given the trend towards ever-larger dental practice organisations though, the two functions of leader and manager are increasingly being split between the owner-dentist(s) who provides the leadership and a practice manager who is employed to administer or manage the practice. With this distinction in mind, let's explore the various differences between leadership and management.

Leaders versus managers

- Managers think incrementally, whereas leaders think radically.
- Managers do things right, leaders do the right thing.
- Managers tend to do things by the book and follow company policy, while leaders follow their own intuition.
- The manager rules; the leader inspires. The manager uses a formal, rational method while the leader lets vision, strategies, goals and values guide actions and behaviour, rather than attempting to control others.
- Managers know how things work but might lack leadership qualities. Leaders may have little or no organisational skills, but their vision unites people behind them.
- Leaders tend to be more emotional than managers. Many believe that people are ultimately governed more by their emotions than their intelligence (their heart rather than their minds) and this explains why teams usually choose to follow leaders.

The net result of these differences is that groups are often more loyal to a leader than to a manager. This loyalty is furthered by the leader taking responsibility in areas such as:

- taking the blame when things go wrong
- celebrating group achievements, even minor ones
- giving credit where it is due.

Successful practitioners realise the importance of being good leaders. Without effective leadership it is difficult to focus and motivate staff members to achieve goals and objectives – not only those of the practice but also their own individual aims. Leadership also involves being accountable and responsible for the group as a whole. Ideally, a leader should be a few steps ahead of the team, but not so far ahead that the team is not able to understand and follow the leader. In short:

> Leaders stand out by being different. They question assumption and are suspicious of tradition. They seek out the truth and make decisions based on fact, not prejudice. They have a preference for innovation. They are sensitive and observant people. They know their team and develop mutual confidence within it. [10]

Leaders need to possess and use a wide range of skills, techniques and strategies. We have already established that you need to articulate your vision so that you yourself can understand where you want to be in the future. During this process we hope that you will have identified those underlying core values that help to shape your mission and, consequently, the way the practice is run. Clearly, you must then be able to communicate your vision to all the members of your team. Failure to do so will make it difficult, if not impossible, to gain the support and enthusiasm necessary to turn this vision into reality. Furthermore, you must not only 'talk the talk' but also 'walk the walk'. In an article appearing in the *Harvard Business Review*, Tony Simons[11] showed how organisations where employees strongly believed their managers followed through on promises and demonstrated the values they preached were substantially more profitable than those whose managers scored average or lower. You set the example for others to follow. To a very large extent, team members and patients alike mimic your behaviour. As Paddi Lund[8] says: 'Politeness is the oil of the wheels of society. It is even more important between married people than strangers.' If you are courteous and gracious in your actions then it is likely they will be in return. 'Treat others as you would wish to be treated yourself' – an old saying but one that has endured because of its simple truth.

WHAT TYPE OF LEADER ARE YOU?

It is possible to look upon leadership as the following sequence of events:
- vision
  ⇓
- planning
  ⇓
- communication
  ⇓
- setting an example
  ⇓
- review.

Establishing your vision was discussed in Strategy 1 and is an essential prerequisite of successful team management. Without knowing where you want to go, how can you expect others to follow with any degree of enthusiasm or commitment? Planning was the subject of Strategy 2 and involves the setting up of systems that allow you to delegate responsibility and permit you to focus 80% of your efforts on your unique ability. The way that you address the twin issues of communicating your vision and establishing a style that sets an example to the rest of the team is a true test of your leadership style. There is no one best way to lead and each approach has its own set of good, and not-so-good, characteristics. With this in mind, which one of the following do you think most closely represents your way of doing things? It would be interesting too to find out which one your staff think comes closest!

The autocrat

The autocratic leader dominates team members to achieve a singular objective. This approach to leadership generally results in passive resistance from team members and requires continual pressure and direction from the leader in order to get things done. Generally, an authoritarian approach is not a good way to get the best performance from a team. There are, however, instances where an autocratic style of leadership may be appropriate. Some situations may call for urgent action, and in these cases an autocratic style of leadership may be best. In addition, most people are familiar with autocratic leadership and therefore have less trouble adopting that style. Furthermore, in some situations, subordinates may actually prefer an autocratic style.

The *laissez-faire* leader

The *laissez-faire* leader exercises little control over his team, leaving them to sort out their roles and tackle their work, without actually participating in this process. In general, this approach leaves the team floundering with little direction or motivation. Again there are situations where the *laissez-faire* approach can be effective but usually only when leading a team of highly motivated and skilled people who have produced excellent work in the past. Once a leader has established that his team is confident, capable and motivated, it is often best to step back and let them get on with the task, since interfering can generate resentment and detract from their effectiveness.

The democrat

The democratic leader makes decisions by consulting the rest of his staff, while still maintaining control of the group. The democratic leader allows the team to decide how tasks will be tackled and who will perform which task. The democratic leader can be seen in two lights. The good democratic leader encourages participation and delegates wisely, but never loses sight of the fact that he bears the crucial responsibility of leadership. He or she values group discussion and input from the rest of the team in order to obtain the best performance. The team is guided with a loose rein and members are motivated and empowered to direct themselves. However, the democrat can also be seen as being so unsure of himself and his relationship with his subordinates that everything is a matter for group discussion and decision. Staff may feel that this type of leader is not really leading at all.

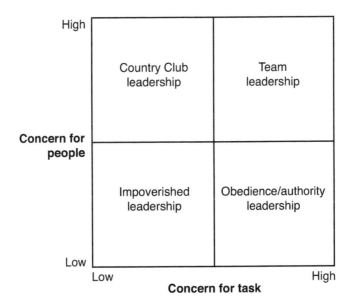

FIGURE 5.2 The way you express your concern for tasks and for people determine your style of leadership

Taking this assessment of your approach a little further, another way of looking at leadership styles is in terms of your:

> *task orientation* – this reflects how much you as a leader are concerned with the various tasks at hand and ensuring that those following you complete them

versus your:

> *employee orientation* – this reflects how much you as a leader are concerned for the people in your team, providing support and encouragement for them.

The combination of these two effects leads to the diagram shown in Figure 5.2. This diagram can be used as a guide to how effective your leadership style is, as your general attitude to leadership will fall into one of these categories. It can also be used as a guide as to how best to lead different individuals using different styles to make the most efficient use of both their and your time and talents.

Impoverished leadership (low concern for task, low concern for people)
This style is characterised by minimal effort on your part, just enough to get the job done and maintain the team.

> *I'll just let them get on with it, I'm sure they are doing fine, they don't really want me interfering anyway.*

Country club leadership (low concern for the task, high concern for people)
You take good care of your group, ensuring a comfortable friendly atmosphere. You hope this will lead to the work getting done. Think of David Brent in the BBC TV series *The Office* and you have the perfect amalgamation of impoverished and country club leadership – someone who confuses popularity with respect:

> *It's obvious – they're happy, they'll work harder and the work will take care of itself.*

Authority/obedience leadership (high concern for task, low concern for people)
You are probably a bit of a taskmaster. The most important thing is the work. You lead from behind by driving the group in front of you. Basil Fawlty probably fits this description.

> *We're here to work, the work needs to be done. If they're working hard enough they won't have time to feel unhappy. After all they're not here to enjoy themselves.*

Team leadership (high concern for task, high concern for people)

You see the completion of the task and the well-being of the group as being interdependent by virtue of you both having a common stake in the organisation's future. This leads to relationships built on trust and respect, and work accomplishment from committed employees. Head of Sky Cycling Sir Dave Brailsford is a fine example of this style of leadership.

> *We're in this together. We need to support and help each other to get this job done.*

Not surprisingly, it is generally accepted that leaders who adopt a team management style are usually the most effective, although this isn't always the case, and choosing the most appropriate style to match the circumstances (directing, coaching, supporting or delegating) is an important and useful skill.

TACTICS FOR TEAM BUILDING

Leadership style is one thing but style can only get you so far. Let's work through the sequence of events that leads to the holy grail of dental practice – the empowered, motivated, enthusiastic team. As you can see from Figure 5.3, this sequence revolves around our shared values – these are at the core of everything we do.

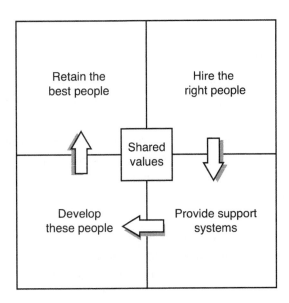

FIGURE 5.3 The team-building cycle

The key question is: *'Do the people in your team feel appreciated?'* In an ideal business environment the following will be the norm:
- the principal appreciates the team and customers
- the team members appreciate the principal, one another and the customers
- customers are selected for their ability to appreciate the team and the principal.

How do you achieve this? Imagine that every human being is like a balloon. Inside the balloon is helium, which represents each person's self-confidence. When you add helium, the balloon expands and rises. Take helium out and the balloon deflates and drops to the ground. Adopt the habit of putting helium into other people's balloons. This is critical. Unless you have a 'helium culture' in place at your business, everything else will be irrelevant. It is the foundation upon which everything works.

Management guru Charles Handy[12] puts it this way:

> *Everyone has a shopping list of what they want from work and life, even if they haven't written it down. The more organisations can match these shopping lists, the more they can expect from their people. Bread-and-butter offerings will elicit bread-and-butter work. Listen to what people really want and give it to them. No-one will be disappointed – organisations that bubble with every type of 'E' (for example, excitement, effort, enthusiasm and energy) are fun to be in.*

THE HELIUM GAME

For the next week, try playing the helium game devised by Dan Sullivan (*see* www.strategic coach.com).[13] Find a way to say or do something to another human being that increases the amount of helium, or self-confidence, that he or she has. It could be your friends, employees, clients, your family, your bank manager, the person at the check-out in Sainsbury's – even the person who cuts in front of you in their car. Why is this important?
- It makes you an extremely 'attractive' person.
- People will be drawn to you.
- Opportunity will be drawn towards you.
- Your own self-confidence will increase as a result.
- The atmosphere in your business will improve dramatically.
- Negative people will naturally move on and leave the business.

As the week progresses make a note, each day, of anyone you consciously added helium to:

Monday

Tuesday

Wednesday

Thursday

Friday

Saturday

Sunday

Did this exercise change your perceptions at all?
Write any comments here:

In order to guide you through the process of building a championship support team we recommend you follow the following nine-step sequence:
1. *eliminate* negative, miserable and incompetent employees
2. *fabricate* an organisational structure
3. *orchestrate* systems for everything
4. *motivate*: recruit, train, motivate and retain your team
5. *indoctrinate*: share your vision with your team
6. *delegate* as much as you possibly can, except the responsibility!
7. *congregate*: make it a priority to listen to your team regularly
8. *compensate* your team well and institute a group performance bonus system
9. *educate*: develop the skills of your team.

Step 1: Eliminate negative, miserable and incompetent employees

How to recruit the right employees

It's not the people you fire that cause problems, it's the people you do not fire. In other words, be as demanding as you can when choosing staff. If you have established a super place to work, where team members are recognised and rewarded and, importantly, are expected to provide a five-star service, then you can afford to be, in fact you *must* be, picky.

The first step in the hiring process is to decide just what type of person you are looking for – a step that is often, amazingly, completely overlooked. You should definitely involve the rest of your team in this task – remember you are trying to find someone who possesses not only whatever technical skills you require but also the beliefs and attitudes that will gel with those of you and your team. Some dentists believe, for example, that prior experience working in another dental practice can be counterproductive in that there may exist attitudes to dentistry that cannot easily be 'de-programmed'. Better, the argument goes, to simply start with a fresh palette and train the person in the skills required.

How do you find these people? Instead of using employment agencies, it can be more effective to use your current contacts and network to find a new member of staff through personal referral. All you need to do is write to people you know to ask them for their help in recommending suitable candidates for the position.

The following is a sample letter you can send to your current database of suppliers, existing staff and clients:

Dear _____

An opportunity for someone you know

As a result of the continuing expansion of the practice, we now have a number of vacancies within our support team.

My reason for writing is to ask whether you know of an individual who could benefit from an employment opportunity at our practice along the following lines:
- here follows the description of the job
- here follows the description of the type of person suitable.

If you are aware of somebody who would be interested in an initial interview then please complete the enclosed sheet giving details of their name, address and telephone number and return it in the reply-paid envelope enclosed.

May I take this opportunity of thanking you for your help in building our business and improving our customer care.

Kind regards

As for the specific job and 'person type' descriptions, how about these two Michael Gerber-inspired examples:[14]

- Wanted: people with passion, people with heart.
- Have you ever wished you could work with a professional business, with professional people, doing professional things in a professional way?
- Well now you can. We are XYZ and we can change the lives of our clients by what we do.
- We are looking for help, for people with a mission.
- No experience is necessary because we will teach you all you need to know.
- But you had better call fast, because we are on a fast track and we're looking for runners.

The purpose of this letter is to get you to contact me. You see, at the moment, I have no idea what your name is but I do know the sort of person you are and I know the aspirations that you have in life.

- I also know the level of skill that you have and that you want to get better and better at your work.
- I know that you want more than a job; you want a career.
- I know that you want more training and you want to have the opportunity to develop a wide range of skills.
- I know that when you call me you will be able to communicate effectively and when we are talking you will be able to discuss important things such as what you can expect from us, as well as things such as your remuneration and your career opportunities.
- I know that you may have had some experience or completed your technical training but, above all, I know that you will have a driving ambition to be the best.
- By the way, this is a permanent position with a talented team of people.
- Please contact me at XYZ.

The interview

The interview itself is not simply a means of finding out specific factual information. It should be built around open-ended questions that assist you in discovering more about the candidate's beliefs and attitudes as well as his or her ability to relate to other people. For example:

- What did you like best about your last job?

- Why did you leave your last job?
- What do you consider most important when working with patients?
- Describe how you handle an angry or difficult patient.
- What have you done at work that you feel especially proud of?
- Why do you feel you can do well in this job?

The interview should help you decide if, and how much, you can trust a particular person. There are three types of trust:
1. *direct trust* – someone you know personally
2. *intuitive trust* – someone your intuition tells you is OK
3. *third-party trust* – someone else knows them and can vouch for them.

This is a valuable yardstick to use when interviewing prospective clients or when interviewing prospective new staff members. Ask yourself these questions:
- What evidence do I have that I can trust, respect and like this person?
- Do I respect what this person has told me about him- or herself – both professionally and personally?
- Do I like being in the same room as this person?

Step 2: Fabricate an organisational structure

Create your organisational structure *first* and then look at the people you have available to fill the positions. What does the structure look like for your business?

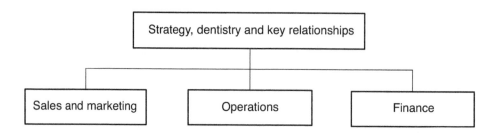

Step 3: Orchestrate systems for everything

In your business do you have systems for:
- answering the phone
- greeting patients
- organising your database
- confirming appointments
- dealing with missed appointments
- selling treatment plans

- follow-up after treatment
- standard letters?

Creating systems for your business takes time but will ultimately save you many hundreds of hours.
- Use your buffer days to spend time on this – *do* it!
- Decide what you need and design a system for it.
- Write it down – create a procedures manual if necessary.
- Make sure the systems are simple and useable.
- Teach your team how to use them.

Systems clarify the exact roles and responsibilities that each team member will play, both individually and as part of the practice team. You need to structure your team in such a way as to provide clear paths of action and responsibility within the group. Overlap or duplication means confusion. For example, a professional approach dictates that all jobs within the practice should have properly designed job descriptions that clearly articulate the following:
- the purpose of the job
- an explanation of the person's duties
- the general working conditions
- how the job relates to those of other members of staff
- the technical and service standards that apply to this job.

Technical standards tend to be the easiest to write, simply because they are the most tangible and, accordingly, the easiest to comply with. Thus, protocols for such activities as developing radiographs, sterilising instruments and backing up computer records are relatively straightforward to compile and, indeed, form the basis of the practice's clinical governance. More difficult to put together, to comply with and, ultimately, to monitor are those standards that reflect the softer, more intangible, aspects of dental practice – for example, ambience, attitudes, empathy, communication, inspiring trust and confidence, and so on. One of the most considered approaches to this whole area is the 'courtesy system' devised by Paddi Lund.[8] While the elements of this system are encapsulated in the following eight performance standards, to gain a better understanding of this system, we strongly recommend that you read Paddi's inspirational book *Building the Happiness-Centred Business*.
1. Blame a system and not a person.
2. Tell the truth.
3. Speak very politely using a person's name – 'please' and 'thank you' as a minimum.

4. When you talk about a person who is not present, speak as if he or she were listening to your conversation.
5. If you have a problem with someone, talk about the problem only with him or her, and in private.
6. Apologise and make restitution if someone is upset by your actions.
7. Greet and say farewell to everyone by name, with eye contact and a touch.
8. Use positive conversation.

Being part of a programme such the well-known 'Investors in People' will force you to create systems that ensure the smooth running of your business. In addition, mind-mapping software such as that provided by Ygnius is a quick and easy way to create your own systems manual.[15]

Make a list here of all the procedures in your business that need to be systemised – and then add a target date by which time you will have developed the system:

Target date
1.
2.
3.
4.
5.
6.
7.

Step 4: Motivate – recruit, train, motivate and retain your team

Question: How do you motivate your team?
Answer: You don't motivate them. Instead you create an environment in which people become self-motivated.

Ensure there is a thriving helium culture in your business
- Live your life as an example to those around you.
- Ensure the people in your team feel fully heard (*see* Step 7: Congregate).

- Be sensitive to the possibility of 'interdepartmental rivalries'. Be open-handed equally and avoid partiality to individuals in your team.
- Avoid the temptation to complain to colleagues or apportion blame when all is not well. This is not the way to build a cohesive and supportive team. Remember, systems are to blame, not people.
- Don't hide in your office in splendid isolation. Communicate openly with the team at all times. Hold regular team meetings that are productive and meaningful and where all team members attend and contribute.
- Encourage and strive for mutual respect between team members.
- Declare an 'amnesty' on mistakes. Tim Kemp[9] recommends that you ask people to note down their 'biggest mistake' while at work. One by one (and starting with you), talk about each instance and let people explore the learning that emerged. Don't expect people to choose their worst clanger the first time you do this activity. Trust needs to be built up over time.

Step 5: Indoctrinate – share your vision with your team

If you have got this far in this book then you will know how much importance we attach to what the first President Bush called 'the vision thing'. Here are a few thoughts to help you share your vision.

- Does your business have a mission statement? Did your employees help you to create it?
- Do your employees have an idea of what the mission statement says?
- Have you shared your vision for your business with your support team?
- How do you intend to do this?
- When do you intend to do this?

Step 6: Delegate as much as you possibly can, except the responsibility

Remember the 80/20 rule:

- 80% of your time is spent on activities that produce 20% of the results
- 20% of your time is spent on activities that produce 80% of the results.

What you must consider is how you can delegate effectively, so that a higher percentage of your time is spent producing top results.

As a business principal you should be spending *80% of your time*:

- developing relationships with the right type of people – suppliers, team, strategic alliances, clients
- helping those people to identify and solve their problems
- asking those people to recommend you to others

and *20% of your time*:

- managing and leading the people to whom you have delegated everything else.

BOX 5.1 Signs that your delegation is failing

- Staff motivation and morale are low.
- You are always working late.
- Your staff are often irritable and the practice atmosphere is tense.
- You get questions about delegated tasks too often.

Not delegating a task because you think that you would do it better than anyone else is a poor excuse. Doing this just makes life difficult for yourself.

How to delegate
- Plan which tasks need to be delegated.
- Identify a suitable person for the task.
- Prepare the person. Explain the task clearly. Make sure that you are understood. Leave some room in the task description for ingenuity and initiative.
- Make sure the person has the necessary authority to do the job properly.
- Monitor progress, provide support and make sure things are on track, but don't get too close. Accept alternative approaches.
- Praise and acknowledge a job well done.

Warning: delegate does not mean dump! You are still responsible for making sure that the task is done on time and correctly. If the person fails, you cannot point the finger. You delegated. You may have picked the wrong person for the job.

Tasks you should not delegate
Obviously, there are some aspects of running a practice that are sensitive and should not be delegated. For example:
- money and pricing
- hiring
- firing
- pay issues
- planning.

For the next few days, keep notes on all the things you do during your workday. How many of these things could you delegate to members of your team?

Activity   Can I delegate this?   Who can I delegate to?

Step 7: Congregate – make it a priority to listen to your team regularly

Group congregation

Take quarterly time out for team meetings. These should last for at least three hours and should be facilitated as a group discussion. This is an opportunity to discuss and review:

- the three-year vision
- the 12-month plan
- the 90-day goals for the next quarter.

It is also an opportunity for your team members to give marks out of 10 on how they think the business is doing in the categories finance, sales, marketing, resources and personnel.

One-to-one congregation

Staff appraisals – do this at least once a quarter.

How to conduct personal progress interviews

Make this a friendly, light, non-confrontational exchange. Just be open, honest and straight; make it safe for both parties to communicate anything. Make sure that you acknowledge all answers verbally and in writing. This method ensures that the employee feels fully heard and acknowledged before any constructive criticism is offered.

FIRST:

Tell your employee that you want to spend a few minutes with him or her having a look at how things are progressing and how the employee feels about his or her job at the moment. Then ask the following questions.

- What do you like best about working here?
- What do you like least about working here?
- If you could wave a realistic magic wand, what would you most like to change about working here?
- If we were to supply you with additional training over the next 12 months, in which area would you most like to be trained?

SECOND:

As the responses to these questions are given, listen carefully, acknowledge the answers, ask for more information if necessary, clarify that you have fully understood your employee's comments and then discuss any actions that may be necessary to build on the good and change the bad.

THIRD:

Explain that you would like to offer some constructive feedback on his or her performance. This takes the following form.

- This is what I like best about your work performance and behaviour.
- This is what I like least about your work performance and behaviour.
- These are the things I would like you to change.

A formal analysis of a team member's hopes and aspirations on a regular basis will stabilise the team member in his or her position and give you early warning if the team member is unhappy with any aspect of his or her place in the team.

Step 8: Compensate your team well and institute a group performance bonus system

People go to work for the following reasons:

- to make money
- to be appreciated
- to have some fun
- to work in a nourishing environment.

To make sure that your team members remain happy, motivated and loyal, follow these four simple steps.

1. Pay them the right money, which means a good competitive wage that is

above average for the geographical or sector position of the business (i.e. top end of basic).

2. Give your staff a guarantee that their basic wage will be reviewed annually in line with average earnings.

3. Implement a group performance-related bonus system. Introduce an element of pay for everyone that is linked to the performance of the business/ organisation as a whole. Create a system whereby, given the achievement of an agreed performance level/target, everybody in the business gets two wage packets in December (i.e. an 8.33% bonus).

4. Be imaginative in thinking of non-financial ways to compensate your staff. For example, consider flexi-time arrangements for assistants or technicians with family responsibilities. People work their best if they are not worrying about neglecting some other aspect of their life.

It is vital to communicate the scheme to the team, and you have to have a means by which everyone can check performance against target. In the staff room you may want to have a graph or a thermometer that shows in an instant how the business is performing against target.

Checklist	Target date	Done
I have communicated my vision and targets fully to the team		✓
I have ensured that they understand the group performance-related bonus scheme		✓
Everyone is clear as to the targets for the business and/or their individual targets		✓
Graph/thermometer is installed in the staff room		✓

Step 9: Educate – develop the skills of your team

It is your responsibility to train your team to do their job better by means of the following.

Training courses

The strength of every team is only as great as its weakest link. All your team members should be encouraged to undergo regular training and professional development. You should invest in your team's future, as well as your own, by facilitating further professional or educational qualifications – the more you put in the more you will get back. Training should ensure that the team forges a mutual understanding of the value of your services and the purpose of your practice. You must ensure that everyone understands the concept of value-added service and is consistently striving to 'go the extra mile' for your patients.

Role-play

If sensitively handled, role play can play a key part in significantly improving your team's ability to do their job well. It will also enhance their self-confidence. Look back at the list you made for the systems needed in your business. Now consider how the use of role play could help your team to implement those systems more effectively.

The following are some areas to consider.

- *Telephony*: how are the phones answered? How is your business being portrayed? Is it always consistent?
- *Reception*: how are your clients greeted? How are they handled at each point of contact? Is there a consistent system?
- *Point of sale*: rehearse how you present treatment options and gain consent.

BOX 5.2 Key points about role-playing

- Make sure the principal is involved and participates before anyone else.
- This is an opportunity for everyone to make mistakes – with each other, *not* clients.
- Consider closing the business down for half a day in order to do this without interruptions.
- Consider taking the team away for a weekend where you will have ample time for role-play as well as other recreational activities.

That is a lot of information to digest, but, as we keep saying, you cannot achieve the success you crave without the backing of a super support team, a team that allows you to create the type of environment that will allow them to flourish. It is one big wheel that feeds on success.

REFERENCES

1. Hamric RE. Common traits of the million-dollar practice. *Dent Econ.* 1996; **86**(6): 34–8, 40, 42, passim.
2. Jeffcoat MK. Hire for attitude, train for skill. *J Am Dent Assoc.* 2002; **133**(11): 1468, 1470.
3. Locker D, Burman D, Otchere D. Work-related stress and its predictors among Canadian dental assistants. *Community Dent Oral Epidemiol.* 1989; **17**(5): 263–6.
4. Blinkhorn AS. Stress and the dental team: a qualitative investigation of the causes of stress in general dental practice. *Dent Update.* 1992; **19**(9): 385–7.
5. Humphris GM, Peacock L. Occupational stress and job satisfaction in the community dental service of north Wales: a pilot study. *Community Dent Health.* 1993; **10**(1): 73–82.
6. Craven RC, Blinkhorn AS, Roberts C. A survey of job stress and job satisfaction among DSAs in the north-west of England. *Br Dent J.* 1995; **178**: 101–4.
7. Mindak MT. Service quality in dentistry: the role of the dental nurse. *Br Dent J.* 1996; **181**(10): 363–8.
8. Lund P. *Building the Happiness-Centred Business.* Capalaba, Australia: Solutions Press; 1994.
9. Kemp T. *The Lonely Practice.* London: BDJ Books; 1994.
10. Fenton J. *101 Ways to Boost Your Business Performance.* Oxford: Heinemann; 1988.
11. Simons T. The high cost of lost trust. *Harv Bus Rev.* 2002; September: 18–19.
12. Handy C. *Inside Organisations: 21 ideas for managers.* London: Penguin Business; 1999.
13. www.strategiccoach.com
14. Gerber M. *The E-Myth Revisited.* New York, NY: Harper Collins; 1995.
15. www.mindgenius.com

FURTHER READING

● Covey S. *Principle-Centred Leadership.* London: Simon & Schuster; 1999.
● Goffee R, Jones G. *Why Should Anyone Be Led By You? What it takes to be an automatic leader.* Boston, MA: Harvard Business School Press; 2006.
● Jaworski J. *Synchronicity: The inner path of leadership.* San Francisco, CA: Berrett-Koehler Publishers; 2011.
● Morrell M, Stephenson A. *Shackleton's Way.* Harmondsworth: Penguin; 2003.
● Morris T. *If Aristotle Ran General Motors.* New York, NY: Henry Holt; 1998.

CHAPTER SIX

Strategy 5: Deliver world-class customer service

You should think of your customers as partners, or better still, family.

Victor Kiam

In recent years 'customer service' has become one of the most prominent business catchphrases, with just about every company these days proclaiming to be customer-focused. As the cover of Ken Blanchard's book on the subject proclaims:

Satisfied customers just aren't good enough. What you need are Raving Fans![1]

Developing such a service-oriented focus, though, demands some understanding and appreciation of your clients' perceptions, attitudes, expectations and desires so that you are in a position to design and tailor the service you offer. Think back to your days as an undergraduate student. Do you remember teachers telling you that the school's aim was to make you *'think like dentists'* . . . perhaps they should have also added that you should just as importantly: *'think like patients'*. The business logic for getting closer to your clients is well established. In a nutshell, satisfied patients are more loyal and spread positive word of mouth to friends, workmates and relatives, whereas dissatisfied customers display little or no loyalty and, even worse, are quite likely to spread negative word of mouth. There is little doubt that bad news travels faster and further than good news. For good news to travel as far, it has to be exceptionally good! If proof were ever needed of this, just think of the number of times you have seen a story in the press about an individual's good experience at the dentist compared with the number of articles dealing with bad experiences. For us dentists, another positive aspect of having happy, satisfied patients is that they tend to be more compliant, more likely to follow our advice and, in the process, make treatment outcomes that bit more predictable.

Satisfying the needs and wishes of our patients ethically and profitably should be one of the most basic goals for any dental practice. Satisfied patients don't just happen though, and the strategies described in this section of the book will help you develop and deliver a range of high-class products and services.

IDENTIFYING WHAT PATIENTS NEED, WANT AND EXPECT

Any service organisation committed to maximising patient satisfaction must come to know its customers and know them well, both collectively and individually. It often seems that, in the case of some dentists, this process happens almost intuitively. Such individuals seemingly possess the ability to understand what people want, even anticipating needs that have not yet been expressed. This impression can be misleading though, since such intuition is usually reinforced by a more considered approach – to such an extent that most highly patient-focused practices are characterised by the ongoing collection of information through activities such as satisfaction surveys and patient interviews. Of course, collection doesn't automatically ensure comprehension, and for such activities to be worthwhile at least an equal amount of attention has to be paid to trying to understand the true meaning behind patients' comments. This is why an increasing number of progressive practices are using more qualitative methods of information gathering (such as questionnaires incorporating open-ended questions and even focus groups) because they allow patients more scope to express their views. Once you start to understand what patients want, it makes sense to try to assess which aspects of the practice are working and which are not. It has been said that the definition of insanity is doing the same thing and expecting a different result. So stop doing what is not working and look for something new to do.

THE MARKETING MIX: WHAT YOU ARE OFFERING YOUR PATIENTS

The marketing mix, commonly referred to as the four 'P's (product, place, price and promotion) is, in effect, an action-oriented framework tailored to communicate to patients information about your services, to ensure they offer value and to make sure they are accessible and convenient. In the case of dental practice, the *product* can be seen as the range of services and products being offered to the patient; *price* is the cost to the patient; the *place* is obviously the practice location in which those services are provided; and, finally, *promotion* encompasses those activities designed to make people aware of the practice and the services offered. Price and promotion are dealt with in Strategies 3 and 7, respectively, but here we will focus on the nature of the product itself and the environment within which that product is delivered to the client.

Conventional wisdom holds that one of the keys to success in business is a successfully implemented marketing mix. It has become clear in recent years, however, that while this philosophy might be appropriate for enterprises such as car dealerships and supermarkets, it fits less easily with those business sectors where the 'product' is much less tangible and much more service-oriented, of which dentistry is clearly a prime example. When we think about dentistry, what exactly is the 'product' we are offering our patients? Is it the actual crown we cement, the denture we place? Or is it in fact something altogether more intangible, such as a sense of well-being? Is it the long-lasting benefit that comes from a relationship built upon the feeling that we really care for our patients and that we have their best interests at heart? Scott MacStravic[2] offered the following thoughts on this subject:

> This 'product' is far different from that of most services, whose long-term impact is typically modest or even non-existent. How long do the benefits of a visit to McDonald's or the local movie theatre last for most people? On the other hand, how much difference can successful medical/surgical care, early detection, health promotion, disease/injury prevention make to patients and families.

This suggests that in order to reach our patients better, we should move away from the traditional view of dentistry (which tends to focus on the treatment itself) and instead concentrate more on communicating the various benefits of care. Patient satisfaction is the result of an evaluation process in which the individual assesses a number of factors. Many of these factors are unrelated to any treatment provided – primarily because most patients do not feel that they possess the necessary knowledge and understanding to make appropriate technical and objective judgements, even after the treatment has been carried out. The truth of the matter is that while the vast majority of patients *do* understand the benefits of being able to chew, of an aesthetic smile and of a freedom from pain and discomfort, they *don't* really understand much about the actual treatment provided, don't even want to understand too much about it and, in most cases, cannot make head nor tail of the jargon we dentists tend to use when talking to them.

Conversely, we all know that the relief of pain and a comfortable, functional and aesthetic result do not necessarily indicate long-term treatment quality. If you are reading this, presumably you know at least a little more about dentistry than the average man in the street – imagine then you have just undergone root canal treatment. How do you know if it is any good or not? The tooth may look and feel fine, but without access to post-operative radiographs how can you be sure that that the canal has been correctly shaped and properly obturated? You cannot, and if you cannot, then imagine the difficulty an average patient would have in making such an assessment. The same can be said for just about every type of treatment we provide. How can a patient know if all subgingival calculus has been removed, or all the caries has been removed from a cavity? How can he or she even know if a restoration was required in the first place?

Because patients cannot easily verify the quality of or even the need for dental treatment, is it surprising then that they are concerned about finding themselves at either end of a continuum characterised by supervised neglect at one end and over-treatment at the other. Clearly, the situation can be extremely confusing for patients – especially when the media is awash with reporters visiting different dentists and receiving a wide variety of advice, treatment plans and fees. In his investigative article 'Can You Trust Your Dentist?', *Reader's Digest* staff writer Tony Dawe[3] reported:

> *Three months and 25 examinations later, I concluded that going to the dentist is nothing to smile about. Dentistry is a stunningly inexact science. Even though I'd expected that different dentists would have different, yet valid, opinions, I was not prepared for the astounding variation in diagnoses I received. One gave me a clean bill of health. Another quoted me £430 for dealing with two teeth and a scale and polish. A third suggested treatment costing £1000 plus. Surely they could not all be right?*

A study of variation in dentists' clinical decisions, carried out in 1995 by James Bader and Daniel Shugars,[4] described such differences as being 'ubiquitous'. They are, however, commonly accepted by the profession as reflections of the natural variation in the best clinical judgement of individual dentists concerning individual patients – the so-called 'art of dentistry'. The only problem, and it is a huge one that must be confronted by the profession, is that such differences in opinion tend to breed mistrust in the public at large who, unsurprisingly, wonder what on earth is going on. Only by fully communicating the various treatment options to our patients and by spending time talking to them about the pros and cons of each approach can we be begin to defuse such mistrust. Critically, we must explain treatment to them in words and terms they do understand, pointing out the benefits that treatment holds for them: 'You will be able to chew better, the surfaces of your teeth will feel so much smoother, you won't show any metal'. Avoid jargon at all costs. Not everyone knows what mastication is or even a crown margin.

Even then, patients will often say something like: 'I'll leave it up to you, doctor – you know best.' Adopting such a paternalistic approach seems an easy way out for the dentist but should be avoided. Wherever possible the patient should be actively involved in the planning process, partly as a courtesy and partly so that the patient feels he or she has a say in how things will be done, a sense of 'ownership' of his or her dental care.

Problems can, of course, also arise in the relatively small number of patients who hold what we might consider to be unrealistic expectations. We are all aware of occasions when we have provided what would generally be considered excellent treatment but which nevertheless fails to satisfy the patient. Dentures are an obvious example. Getting close to the patient means understanding their expectations before treatment begins. Although we might dearly wish to fulfil all our patient's expectations, trying to do so in the patient with unrealistic demands usually courts disaster, as common sense and fundamental principles often end up being ignored. It is important to stress though that so-called body dysmorphic disorder[5] does not play a significant role in the majority of people who seek cosmetic dental care. Research carried out in Holland found that only one of the characteristics of body dysmorphic disorder – namely, a preoccupation with a defect of appearance – emerged as a significant predictor of the desire to undergo cosmetic dental treatment.[6] This research found that patients with such preoccupation were nine times more likely to consider tooth whitening and six times more likely to consider orthodontic treatment. Significantly, they were also five times more likely to be dissatisfied with their most recent treatment.

Understanding full well their own limitations when it comes to making value judgements on the quality of work provided, the vast majority of patients just want to feel they can place their trust in us and feel confident that we will take care of them. Is this so difficult to believe? Think about the times you fly off to that holiday in the sun. Do you really want to know the technical ins and outs of how the pilot is going to fly the plane? Probably not. By getting on the plane you have put your trust in the airline and to be honest you are far more likely to be interested in the quality of service provided in the cabin, whether you take off and arrive on time, and so on, rather than worrying if the pilot knows what lever to pull.

These simple truths were borne out by one study conducted at the Marquette University School of Dentistry in Milwaukee.[7] The results of the study indicated that no relationship existed between the quality measures used by patients and dentists. The authors concluded that patients and dentists were studying different criteria when they considered quality and that

> *simply practicing dentistry with a high degree of technical expertise will not necessarily convince the patient that he or she has received high-quality dental care. Other less technical aspects of dental treatment are recognised by the patient as being barometers of quality of dental treatment.*[7]

If patients feel that their assessments of technical quality are not valid then what do they use as the basis for their judgements? Put simply, they use those aspects of care that they do understand and about which they do feel capable of holding opinions. For example:

- *Care* – was I made to feel that I was their number one priority?
- *Courtesy* – was I treated fairly and with respect?
- *Communication* – was everything fully explained to me?
- *Comfort* – was the treatment painful or uncomfortable?
- *Cost* – did I receive value for money?
- *Convenience* – could I organise my visits at times that were convenient for me?
- *Cues* – what do I think of the physical evidence of service?

Thus, most patients do have a very clear understanding of how they are treated as people. This is of fundamental importance to them but, as Redford and Gift[8] discovered, dentists tend to be more adept at describing patients in terms of dental conditions and/or treatment needs than personal characteristics:

> *I think she was the one that had that lower right molar in tough shape – endo, perio . . . just a real mess.*

or

> *I was concentrating more on the teeth and not paying as much attention to the person.*

Patients know all too well when they are not being respected or are being treated in a less than caring way, when they are not being listened to, or their views not considered. It is painfully obvious when practice staff are flustered or arguing with each other or seem to be so involved in other things to the extent that the patient is far from being what he or she should be, the very centre of everyone's attention.

Patients notice if the practice *feels* unprofessional. In fact, professionalism is one of things that is difficult to describe but you certainly know it when you see it, and equally you notice when it is absent. Patients are no longer going to tolerate the conditions that exist in many practices. I am sure we have all seen house-proud patients running their finger along the dental light and have cringed when they find that speck of dust that tells them more about us than any perfectly executed cavo-surface angle ever could. Professionalism is a heady cocktail of the tangible and the intangible, and when present it instils a confidence and trust in patients that sees them putting their faith and mouths in the hands of the dentist. This need of patients to be able to trust the practice is central to our philosophy.

The sad fact, though, is that dentists and their staff often seriously misjudge the way that they are evaluated by patients, with the result that too much effort is put into areas that don't really influence the patient's thinking instead of those aspects of practice that do – for example, trying to explain to patients the intricacies of tangible items of equipment such as computers or lasers (all of which fascinate the dentist but hold less interest to the patient) instead of showing real concern for the patient's fears and anxieties.[9] One study that compared criteria of 'good practice' as proposed by on the one hand dentists and on the other, patients, suggested that dentists believe they know what patients should want, rather than finding out what they do want.[10] In a similar vein, another study described the psychological trauma many patients undergo during and after tooth extraction, ranging from a real dislike of having to sit in the dental chair without their denture(s) to the sense of bereavement felt when teeth are lost.[11] The implications are that dentists and their staff should spend at least as much time understanding and concentrating on such patient-oriented issues as they perhaps do trying to explain about those aspects of care that are of little or no meaning to the patient.

THE PATIENT JOURNEY

Your patient's trust and confidence doesn't happen with a single, solitary act, no matter how amazing that may be. Instead, it is built by providing regular and often unspectacular consistency, one step at a time. Each step is one of Jan Carlzon's '*moments of truth*' in which your goal should be to deliver what you promise, how you promised it and to do so consistently.[12] These steps come together to make a patient journey that begins long before you, as the dentist, get to meet the patient and hopefully never really ends. Your aim should be for your clients *and* your staff to have an exceptional experience whenever they are in your business premises. What is the perfect patient journey? A series of

12 steps, to be learned by principals and teams, to ensure world-class customer service, every time (*see* Box 6.1).

BOX 6.1 The patient journey

- The telephone enquiry and/or first visit
- The pre-first appointment paperwork
- The arrival at the reception
- The patient lounge
- The journey to the surgery
- The initial conversation
- The clinical examination
- The treatment-planning discussion
- The treatment plan
- Delivering the treatment
- Back to the reception
- The post-visit action and paperwork

Each of these steps can be adapted to the individual style of your practice and your team. There are no scripts, just a philosophy of offering services.

SYSTEMATIC SPONTANEITY

Have you ever noticed that when people tell you about 'WOW' service they have received, it is usually a gesture that was probably systematic but received as an expression of spontaneous customer service.

Examples are:
- the dentist who gives his patients hot towels after a course of treatment
- the RAC who called you to update you on arrival time after 15 minutes of waiting for a recovery vehicle
- the hotel receptionist who, after telling you that all of his rooms were taken, offered to ring local hotels to find an alternative for you
- the restaurant manager who offered complimentary desserts after a main course was delayed.

The trend is that a pleasant individual took the trouble to make sure you felt really appreciated as a customer – that's why you will keep going back and keep telling all your friends. None of these examples are of the cheapest provider – but people choose to pay 'extra' for the individual attention. So if you have chosen to offer your customers the best, rather than the best price, what 'systems' do you have in place to make sure they are WOWed? Some examples are outlined here.

Telephony

Is there an agreed system by which a prospective new customer is handled on the phone? *Not* a script but an agreed procedure.

Arrival

The customer arrives at the practice. What is his or her experience of being welcomed, given paperwork to fill out, offered refreshments, shown to seat, and so forth?

On-site

The patient lounge: is the customer informed as to how long they will have to wait? Are they further informed of any delays? The customer is shown to the surgery. Are your assistants trained to do this properly? Is there a handshake, a warm smile, an introduction, eye contact, good communication skills?

Departure

The client is escorted from the surgery, back to reception and to the front door. Does the client receive all the information and paperwork he or she needs? Is there a standard procedure for payment and making future appointments?

Post visit

What does the client receive by way of follow-up? A letter or a phone call?

SYSTEMATIC SPONTANEITY SYSTEMS

- Schedule some time for your whole team to take part in this exercise.
- Imagine that you are a customer, travelling through your business and make a list of all the steps in the customer journey.
- Write a list of 10 things that you could do that would demonstrate 'systematic spontaneity'.
- When you have completed this list, ask the team what would have to happen for these systems to be implemented.
- Decide which is going to be your 'flagship WOW' – the one thing that you do that will have people raving about you – tick the relevant box and set a deadline for implementation.

	Our flagship WOW ✓	Deadline
1.	☐	
2.	☐	
3.	☐	
4.	☐	

PHYSICAL FACILITIES

When a customer visits your business:

	✗	✓
What do they see?	Peeling wallpaper, dingy décor, dusty surfaces, outdated magazines	Clean, fresh-looking, pleasant, tasteful décor, fresh flowers
What do they hear?	Gossip, negative comments, noisy equipment, unpleasant music	No gossip, soothing music, laughter
What do they taste?	Cheap tea, instant coffee, tap water	Real coffee, herbal tea, mineral water
What do they smell?	Antiseptic, unpleasant odours	Pleasant, soothing aromas
What do they feel?	Uncomfortable chairs, cheap cups, plastic glasses	Comfortable seats in reception area, smooth surfaces, quality cups and glasses

The WOW practice relates to your team as well as your clients. People will perform better in a nourishing environment. Remember, your aim should be that:

- your customers feel appreciated – by you and your team
- your team feels appreciated – by you, their peers and your customers
- you feel appreciated by your team and your customers.

How close does your practice come to being a WOW practice?

THE WOW PRACTICE

Take a hard look at your physical facilities from cus-tomer's point of view and jot down some notes.

Current reality:

Note your scores (1–10) for each of the five senses in the boxes below

Sight ☐   Sound ☐   Taste ☐   Smell ☐   Feel ☐

What improvements will you make to score a 10?

What could you add that would make a visit to your business truly *outstanding* – an experience that eve-rybody talks about? See the column on the right for some ideas.

- Fresh flowers
- Restful colour scheme
- Good-quality carpet
- Comfortable seats in reception area
- Minimal waiting time
- Lots of natural light
- Minimal chatter
- Soothing music
- Electric automatic aromatherapy
- Coffee machine – cappuccinos offered
- Fresh mineral water
- Well-maintained exterior and entrance
- Friendly, smiling, efficient staff
- Clean, modern treatment rooms
- Tasteful décor
- Original artwork in waiting room
- Follow-up phone call or letter after treatment
- Welcome letter plus directions to practice
- Comfortable temperature
- Hot towels after treatment
- Greet clients by name
- Up-to-date magazines
- Remember small details about customers
- Scrupulously clean, pleasant washroom
- High-quality soaps in washroom
- Scent in washroom
- Fresh hand towels in the washroom

REFERENCES

1. Blanchard K. *Raving Fans! A revolutionary approach to customer service.* New York, NY: Harper Collins; 2011.
2. MacStravic S. The death of the four 'P's: a premature obituary. *Mark Health Serv.* 2000; **20**(4): 16–20.
3. Dawe T. Can you trust your dentist? *Reader's Digest.* 1998; **152**: 50–7.
4. Bader JD, Shugars DA. Variation in dentists' clinical decisions. *J Public Health Dent.* 1995; **55**(3): 181–8.
5. Scott SE, Newton JT. Body dysmorphic disorder and aesthetic dentistry. *Dent Update.* 2011; **38**(2): 112–18.
6. De Jongh A, Oosterink FMD, van Rood YR, *et al.* Preoccupation with one's appearance: a motivating factor for cosmetic dental treatment? *Br Dent J.* 2008; **204**(12): 691–5.
7. Abrams R, Ayers C, Vogt Petterson M. Quality assessment of dental restorations: a comparison by dentists and patients. *Community Dent Oral Epidemiol.* 1986; **14**(6): 317–19.
8. Redford M, Gift HC. Dentist-patient interactions in treatment decision-making: a qualitative study. *J Dent Educ.* 1997; **61**(1): 16–21.
9. Newsome P, Wright G. Qualitative techniques to investigate how patients evaluate dentists: a pilot study. *Community Dent Oral Epidemiol.* 2000; **28**(4): 257–66.
10. Burke L, Croucher R. Criteria of good dental practice generated by general dental practitioners and patients. *Int Dent J.* 1996; **46**(1): 3–9.
11. Fiske J, Davis DM, Frances C, *et al.* The emotional effects of tooth loss in edentulous people. *Br Dent J.* 1998; **184**(2): 90–3.
12. Carlzon J. *Moments of Truth.* Cambridge, MA: Ballinger; 1989.

FURTHER READING

- Lund P. *Building the Happiness-Centred Business.* Capalaba, Australia: Solutions Press; 1994.
- Newsome P. *The Patient-Centred Dental Practice: A practical guide to consumer care.* London: BDJ Books; 2001.

CHAPTER SEVEN

Strategy 6: Refine your selling skills

Any fool can paint a picture, but it takes a wise man to sell it.

Samuel Butler

There are so many misconceptions about selling. It has, for many people, so many negative connotations that they almost recoil at hearing the word. In truth we should see selling as a very sensitive, compassionate, ethical and professional way to help our clients to make decisions.

- *Selling is not* profiteering, browbeating or a gladiatorial contest.
- *Selling is* delivering five-star services or products and helping your clients to purchase them.

There are many definitions of selling, often comparing it with marketing. Take, for example, the following from the late Harvard-based marketing guru Theodore Levitt:

> *Selling focuses on the needs of the seller; marketing on the needs of the buyer. Selling is preoccupied with the seller's need to convert his product into cash; marketing with the idea of satisfying the needs of the customer by means of the product and the whole cluster of things associated with creating, delivering and finally consuming it.*[1]

This definition, and others like it, portrays selling negatively. We, on the other hand, see selling and marketing as being complementary to each other:

- *Marketing*: the process by which you accumulate a reservoir of people who may, one day, be interested in buying.

● *Selling*: the process by which you help a person who is in the reservoir make an informed and well-timed decision to buy.

One of the best comments we have heard on this subject has been attributed to Gabriel Siegel, who wrote:

> *Most salesmen try to take the horse to water and make him drink. Your job is to make the horse thirsty.*

How often do our treatment proposals try to force our clients to drink? What can we do to shape our approach in a way that will make them pant for more?

SELLING: A 20-STEP PROCESS
Steps 1–7: preparing to sell
Step 1: Preparation
You must be mentally prepared before you begin to sell. As Dan Sullivan says, self-confidence is crucial:

> *You cannot achieve anything personally or professionally from a starting position of low self-esteem.*[2]

Once you have the confidence in yourself, then you are able to focus your attention on others. As we have said before, when you are with a client you must believe that he or she is the most important person in the world to you at that moment. To help you get to this state of mind we would like you to think what your life would be like if you could magically wipe the slate clean . . .

A CLEAN SLATE

Date _____

Have you ever wondered what it would be like to start all over again, knowing what you know now – but with a completely clean slate? All of that personal experience, learning and wisdom? None of those complications, legacies, obligations, doubts, limiting beliefs, traditions, tolerations, mistakes? Well now you can . . .

Steps

- Find a quiet place, free from interruption, and schedule some time for yourself.
- Imagine that you are able to change your personal life over the next 90 days, with all of your assets and skills but with none of your liabilities and perceived weaknesses.
- Write a list of the top 10 things that you would do differently, or have differently around you, over the coming 90 days.
- Take time to consider what you have written.
- Ask yourself: '*So what would happen if I did this anyway, made these decisions, requests and put in place these boundaries?*'
- Consider the outcome(s).
- Consider the possibilities of doing things differently anyway!

BUSINESS

1.
2.
3.
4.
5.
6.
7.
8.
9.
10.

PERSONAL

1.
2.
3.
4.
5.
6.
7.
8.
9.
10.

Step 2: Attitude

The reason people don't ask a client to buy is fear of rejection. To sell effectively it is essential to adopt the right attitude to rejection. If someone says 'no', they don't want to buy your product or service, all you have to do is follow these simple steps.

You ask: *Is that no never, or is it no, not now?*
If they say: *'No never'* then just walk away from the conversation and delete them from your reservoir.
If it's: 'No, not now' then say, *'That's fine – tell me when would it be OK for me to make a diary note to contact you again?'*

Step 3: Practice

Practice on others, *not* your clients. Take time out for selling skills training – schedule periods of time to train yourself and your team on selling skills, either in-house or at another location. The use of role-playing is just as useful in selling as it was in Strategies 4 and 5.

Step 4: Create the time to learn to sell and in which to sell

You cannot sell in a rush – be sure to create ample space in which to sell properly. This means lengthening the time invested in routine examinations.

Step 5: Create a menu of all the services you offer

Do your clients understand everything you can do for them? Do they understand how it can benefit them? Your menu should focus on *outcome* first and *method* second. Remember, you are selling benefits.

Make a list of the top 10 products/services that you offer.

1.   6.

2.   7.

3.   8.

4.   9.

5.   10.

Now rewrite this list in terms of how each item benefits the client (e.g. 'Tooth whitening' might become 'A Hollywood smile' or 'A permanent solution to discoloured teeth'). Be sure to write clearly and in language the client can understand – avoid jargon.

1.   6.

2.   7.

3.   8.

4.   9.

5.   10.

You are then ready to compose your own dental menu. Consider the example provided here by Dr Anthony Fagg of the Eastgate Dental Practice.

Top 10 ways we can improve your dental appearance

- If you think your teeth are too dark or discoloured we can lighten them. This is a simple treatment that can be carried out at home, is pain-free and can produce amazing results.
- Unsightly or misshapen teeth can be disguised using veneers to make them blend in with your other teeth.
- Do you have old crowns on your front teeth that do not match your other teeth? We can replace them with natural-looking metal-free porcelain crowns.
- If you have old or stained fillings that are visible when you smile, we can make them almost invisible with tooth-coloured composite restorations.
- Large, old, silver fillings often become unsightly. We can replace them with tooth-coloured composite restorations or porcelain inlays.
- If you have missing teeth the spaces can be filled with bridges or by implants.
- Do you have a denture that looks or feels false? We can, in the majority of cases, produce natural-looking cosmetic dentures for an improved appearance and better bite.
- Are your teeth stained or your gums red and swollen? We can improve the appearance of both by polishing and periodontal treatment.
- If your teeth are twisted, crowded or out of line it is never too late to improve them. We may be able to provide orthodontic treatment (braces) to improve your smile.
- Are the tips of your teeth uneven? Often we can quickly, painlessly and without the need of an anaesthetic recontour or level the tips of your teeth to improve your smile

Top 10 ways we can improve your dental health

- Do your gums bleed when brushing? Do you get a bad taste in your mouth or around some teeth? Do your gums look red or swollen? Modern periodontal treatment will ensure trouble-free healthy gums.
- Are you apprehensive about injections or the drill? Have your fillings done using Carisolv – a new technique that removes decay without the need for an anaesthetic or drilling in most situations.
- Do your teeth keep breaking? We can strengthen them with crowns.
- If you have missing teeth, certain problems can occur (other than the obvious one of spoiling your smile). There may be movement of teeth nearby, which will affect your bite and then possibly the gum health. We can replace missing teeth with bridges and implants.
- Are you unhappy with your old plastic partial denture? We can replace it with a metal-based denture, which will be stronger, tighter, less damaging to your gums and more comfortable to wear.
- Tooth decay is painful and it can be expensive to repair the damage. Decrease your chance of decay with preventive treatment.
- Are your teeth sensitive to cold? Consider desensitising.
- If you play contact sports regularly we can supply a custom-made mouthguard (gum-shield) to protect your teeth.
- If you feel that your teeth do not meet together very well we can improve the effectiveness of your bite with occlusal equilibration.
- We all suffer symptoms of stress. We can reduce headaches and tension pains around the jaws with splints.

Step 6: Develop trust with potential clients

The subject of trust was discussed at length in Strategy 5 and is something that is central to the selling process:

- if you sell products and services with trust you have 'clients' (who develop a relationship with you over many years)
- if you sell products and services without trust you have 'customers' (who buy and leave).

There are three types of trust:

1. *long-term trust*: built through fulfilling promises you have made to people
2. *instinctive trust*: knowing intuitively that someone you meet for the first time is someone you can trust
3. *third-party trust*: someone who is recommended by someone you know who knows and trusts the other person.

Trust is also a two-way thing – for your own part you should never do business with someone you instinctively don't like. Listen to your intuition. If it doesn't feel right, walk away from the deal.

Step 7: Teamwork – selling is a team event

As your clients move through your business premises, each step of the way is part of the selling process – 'The patient journey'. Do you have a system for this? Are your staff trained for the roles they play in the selling process?

 Make a list of every opportunity that could exist in your business for a selling conversation:

Steps 8–17: selling skills

Step 8: Listening

In a sales conversation:

- the *buyer* is the one who should *talk* the most
- the *seller* is the one who should *listen* the most.

Key skills that you must try to develop here are:

- eye contact
- body language
- silence – the most important listening skill of all.

The need for listening is obvious, yet it is difficult to listen well. Listening enables you to understand your patient's perceptions, feel his or her emotions and hear what he or she is trying to say. Active listening improves not only what you hear, but also what the patient says. In their book *Getting to Yes*, Roger Fisher and William Ury[3] say that if you pay attention and interrupt occasionally to say, 'Did I understand correctly that you are saying that . . .?' the other person will feel the satisfaction of being heard and understood. They suggest that you make it your task while listening not to phrase a response but to understand the other person as that person sees him- or herself. Take in the person's perceptions, needs and constraints. It also helps to sit on the same side of a table and to have in front of you the materials you need – this way the time together becomes a side-by-side activity in which the two of you jointly face a common task.

Step 9: Develop empathy with the client

Empathy means putting yourself in the other person's shoes. You must view any given situation through his or her eyes. The ability to see the situation as the other side sees it, as difficult as that may be sometimes, is one of the most important skills you must develop.

- Listen carefully.
- Use silence.
- Mirror the other person's body language.
- Make sure you understand the background to the client's desire for a conversation and the context in which the client is asking.

Step 10: Opening the sales conversation

There are three options:

1. *'How can I help.?'*

   Stop talking and **listen**

2. *'If I could make one wish come true – about how our products/services could help you – what would that wish be?'*

   Stop talking and **listen**

3. *'If I could wave a realistic magic wand, and you could have the perfect outcome of our professional relationship, what would it be?'*

   Stop talking and **listen**

Step 11: Fact-finding

The sort of information you need to gather is of two types:

1. hard facts: name, address, contact details, bank information, clinical assessment
2. soft facts:
   - 'How do you feel about ___?'
   - 'How would it feel if ___?'
   - 'What's really important to you about ___?'

 Write down two to three 'soft-fact' questions that you would feel comfortable using and start incorporating them into your sales conversations.

1.

2.

3.

Step 12: Understand the client's hot buttons

What is the hook that will help to make the client take action? Is there an up-and-coming event in the client's life that could create a deadline or focus for the sale? What do they really need and want. You find the answers to these questions through asking soft fact-finding questions such as those outlined in the previous step.

Step 13: Challenging the client – playing tennis at the net

The sales conversation is very similar to a game of tennis. Imagine that you are playing at the net. You have total control while the person on the other side is running back and forth along the baseline, chasing all the shots.

How do you stay at the net in a sales conversation? *Don't jump into answering questions.* Instead, insist that clients determine the answer themselves. For example:

Client: *'I don't know. That seems very expensive.'*

Instead of running to the baseline and coming up with reasons why your service is such good value for money, *stay at the net* and ask a question, such as:

'What is it about the price that concerns you?'

or

'Could you clarify something for me – are you concerned about the value of the investment or the timing?'

or

'If you could wave a magic wand, how would you want to pay for this service?'

Role-play the tennis game! Stop running to the baseline. Stay at the net!

Step 14: Recognise the moment of truth = the point that the client says 'yes'
If they say *yes*, stop your presentation and sign them up. Even if you haven't finished what *you* want to say, you have finished what *they* want to hear! Due diligence and paperwork can follow later.

Step 15: Give people options
People like choices, so let them have different service choices, different treatment options, different payment options, and so forth. For example, if you give people three choices they are most likely to choose the middle one.
1. Bronze service
2. Silver service
3. Gold service.

If most of your clients are choosing the gold option, then your prices are too low!

Step 16: Dealing with objections
We suggest two key tactics for dealing with (inevitable) misgivings.
1. *Anticipation.* Research and role-play all possible objections. Think why people would say no and rehearse an appropriate response. Build the answers to those objections into the way you present your products and services.
2. *Feel – felt – found.* When a client raises an objection, simply say:

I understand how you feel – you are not the first person who has said that they felt this was a problem. But what I have found in practice is that people who have proceeded to the next level have been happy with the outcome.

Step 17: Closing the sale

When do you do this? When the other person is ready – not when you are. This doesn't have to be complicated. Just ask: *'Is there any reason why we can't get started?'*

- If the response is *yes*, ask what the reason is, and deal with the concerns.
- If the response is *no*, get the paperwork out and sign the deal.
- If they want to *think about it*, talk it over with their spouse, and so forth, that is fine but do not let them off the hook. Stay in control by asking: *'When would you like me to ring you for a decision?'*

Steps 18–20: after the sale

Step 18: Cement the sale

Find some way to follow up. For example:

- *send written confirmation* – a short summary on one side of letterhead, and/or
- *send a thank-you card* – 'I enjoyed meeting you, looking forward to working with you' and so forth.

Step 19: Referrals

Post sale is a good time to ask for referrals.

> *I'm delighted you decided to proceed with my recommendations. Right now is there anyone you would like to receive a copy of our welcome pack?*

Step 20: Après sale – marginal marketing

The following are great ways to add value to clients and get people talking about your unique service (for more of this *see* Strategy 7: Create a low-cost marketing engine):

- birthday cards
- postcards from holiday
- bunch of flowers
- cinema tickets
- good luck cards
- bottle of wine
- clippings service.

REFERENCES

1. Levitt T. Marketing myopia. *Harv Bus Rev.* 1975; September/October: 45–56.
2. www.strategiccoach.com
3. Fisher R, Ury W. *Getting to Yes*. New York, NY: Penguin Books; 1983.

FURTHER READING

- Beckwith H. *Selling the Invisible*. New York: Warner Books; 1997.
- Boress A. *I Hate Selling*. New York: AMACOM; 1995.
- Hopkins T. *Selling for Dummies*. Chichester: John Wiley & Sons; 2001.
- Kline N. *Time to Think*. London: Cassell Illustrated; 1998.
- Mackay H. *Swim with the Sharks without being Eaten Alive*. New York: Ballantine Books; 1996.
- Newsome P, Latter A. *Helping Patients to Say 'Yes': Ethical selling for the dental team*. London: Stephen Hancocks; 2009.
- Seth J, Sobel A. *Clients for Life*. New York: Simon and Schuster; 2000.

CHAPTER EIGHT

Strategy 7: Create a low-cost marketing engine

*All the money that you need for the rest of your career is in the pockets of
the people that you already know and the people they can introduce you to.*

Dan Sullivan

Just as with selling, there are many textbook definitions of marketing, most of
which say something like:

The process by which you attract new customers.

We prefer to define marketing though as:

The process by which you eliminate the customers you don't want.

We also have one ground rule and that is that the objective is to spend as little
money as possible on marketing – don't, however, confuse money with effort
and thought.

Marketing and dentistry go back a long way and the relationship between
the two has been, and in some ways continues to be, quite fraught. For many
dentists the idea that we should go out and promote ourselves seems inappropriate. Just like Molière's Monsieur Jourdain, who was delighted to learn that he
had been speaking prose all his life, every dentist is marketing him- or herself
even when the dentist does not think of him- or herself as doing so. All of us
are sending out messages to our clients that build up a picture in their minds
about who we are, what we stand for and what we provide. We believe that it

makes much more sense to be in control of those signals so that the person receiving them perceives what we want them to perceive, with as little as poss- ible left to chance. One of the most obvious of these signals is your business image, and before considering specific internal and external marketing tactics you must ensure that you have in place the correct business image. Elements of your business image include:

- business name
- logo
- literature
- environment
- strapline.

We approach the subject of marketing by looking at both your internal and external activities.

INTERNAL MARKETING TECHNIQUES

Step 1: Grade your existing clients

Grading is a team event. The team should be involved, as they have to deal with clients as well.

Category 'A' client

Someone who loves you and what you do. Not only can the client spend money with you today but also he or she has the capacity to continue spending money with you for his or her lifetime. The client is also well connected personally or professionally and is at the centre of a network, which means that if you do a good job the client is likely to recommend you to others.

Category 'B' client

Someone who loves you and what you do. However, the client may not be able to spend quite so much money now or in the future, and/or he or she may have a lower level of connectivity.

Category 'C' client

Someone who cannot make his or her mind up about you and/or your prod- ucts and services. The client doesn't respond to letters, doesn't fill in forms, fails to arrive for appointments on a regular basis, and is not committed to having a regular relationship with you. He or she is likely to recommend you to other category 'C' clients. 'C' is for choice – the client must choose whether to become an 'A', a 'B' or a 'D'.

Category 'D' client

The Victor Meldrew/BMW (bitcher, moaner and whiner). 'D' is for delete. Get rid of them. Keep putting up your prices and they will probably go away. If this does not work, you will need to speak to them and suggest other people who can help them.

Category 'SC' client

We all have some clients who we will serve out of a 'social conscience' – they simply cannot afford or can no longer afford our services and yet we want to help. Sometimes this is as a reward for previous loyalty and other times just because we care. This is fine, so long as it represents a small proportion of our time and we are not 'duped' by those who simply don't want to pay.

> **Objective**: To end up with only 'A' and 'B' clients – preferably 20% of As generating 80% of the profit and 80% of Bs generating 20% of the profit.

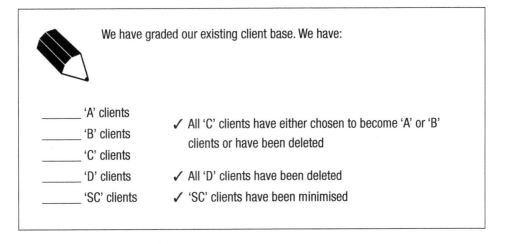

We have graded our existing client base. We have:

_____ 'A' clients

_____ 'B' clients

_____ 'C' clients   ✓ All 'C' clients have either chosen to become 'A' or 'B' clients or have been deleted

_____ 'D' clients   ✓ All 'D' clients have been deleted

_____ 'SC' clients   ✓ 'SC' clients have been minimised

Step 2: Create a menu

How are your new and existing clients given the opportunity of buying more from you? For this to happen, they must be aware of *all* the products and services that are available to them and all the ways that these products and services can benefit them. You need to create a menu of the full range of products and services you have to offer (*see* Strategy 6: Preparing to sell, Step 5, page 120). If you haven't done this, please do it now. If you have, please return to it and review and update as necessary. Once you have created your menu, you need to do something with it! Be proactive.

At some point during the client's journey through the business premises, ensure that somebody presents the menu to the client, asking him or her to take a few minutes to read through it and to tick the subjects in which he or she is interested.

- Include the menu in your practice brochure.
- Include the menu on your website.
- Display the menu somewhere in your reception area.
- Include the menu with your recall letter.
- Include the menu with your end-of-treatment letter.

Make sure the language of the menu is about the clients' outcomes and not your 'mumbo jumbo'.

Step 3: Produce a welcome pack

We believe it is extremely important to provide new clients with a welcome pack. A practical format is a printed folder with a pocket into which you can insert the following:

- mission statement
- practice information leaflet/brochure
- CVs/profiles
- testimonials
- terms and conditions
- promises
- prices
- menu.

Step 4: Develop a referral system

Do you have a system for asking existing clients to refer others to you? When do you ask for referrals?

The first time you make contact with a potential new client

Somewhere in the information you give or send to them include a sentence like this:

> *The bulk of our business comes through personal recommendations. If we do a good job, we would be very happy for you to refer others to us.*

The first time you physically meet a potential new client

Let them know that:

> Most of our new business comes through personal recommendations. We promise you
> certain things – if we do a good job we would like you to refer others to us.

During the selling process

Client: *'How much will it cost?'*

You: *'We get paid in two ways. First, we are paid for the specific service we provide,
and second, if we do a five-star job, we ask you to recommend us to others. Is
that OK with you?'*

At the end of treatment

Write an end-of-treatment letter along the lines of:

> We have now completed this treatment. How was it for you? Any problems please let us
> know. You will recall that our business grows through personal recommendations. Here
> are three copies of our leaflet/brochure/referral card. Please feel free to pass these on to
> anyone else who you think would benefit from our product or service.

In any newsletter or other printed marketing material.

Include referral permission, for example:

> We have vacancies available for the right type of client. Please feel free to recommend
> us to anyone you think would be interested.

If you have a website, it is essential that you have a referral permission statement and the ability to recommend others to your website.

Step 5: Produce a referral card

Your referral card gives people an insight into what you do and what sort of clients you are looking for. Roughly double the size of a business card and printed
on both sides, it should ideally include the following:

- logo
- contact details
- your photo
- description of ideal client
- mini menu of what you offer or an explanation of the main outcomes
  you deliver.

Your referral card can be included with preliminary information, sent with the
end-of-treatment letter and/or handed out at networking events.

EXTERNAL MARKETING TECHNIQUES

Step 1: Build your reservoir

Imagine that all the potential new clients you come into contact with are represented by the water that builds up in a reservoir. The reservoir is built up of people who have said 'No, not now' (*see* Strategy 6). When the reservoir is full, the water begins to trickle over the top. In other words, when you have enough people in your reservoir, by a natural process some of them automatically spill over the top and become ready to buy your products and services.

Your goal should be to create a reservoir system and devote yourself to filling it with 1000 names, making sure that it is continually filled through marketing activities and making sure too that you 'tickle' the people in your reservoir continually. By 'tickling' we mean that you have some system for following up with the people in your reservoir on a regular basis, for example:

- follow-up phone call or email
- newsletter
- tips
- special offers
- newspaper articles.

Step 2: Use networking

Networking is a great way to add more people to your reservoir. To do this you need to get out into the personal and professional world and give as many people as you can your referral card and deliver an effective elevator speech. *See* Box 8.1 for a description of what you can do in 20 seconds, adapted to your own personal style, to attract people and encourage them to want to know more about you and the product or service you provide.

BOX 8.1 Elevator speech

Well you know how some people . . .

- experience: a lack of confidence because their teeth are crooked
- which means that: they don't smile as often as they would like to
- well, what I do is: offer cosmetic dentistry
- the benefit of which is: the teeth can be straightened
- which means that: they are happier because they can smile with confidence.

Would you be interested in knowing more?

Draft your own elevator speech

Well you know how some people . . .
- experience:
- which means that:
- well, what I do is:
- the benefit of which is:
- which means that:

Would you be interested in knowing more?

Where to network
- Chamber of Commerce
- business link
- business breakfast clubs
- business networking groups
- complementary professions
- special interest groups
- golf club
- sports events

Step 3: Public speaking

This is a very effective way of filling your reservoir. It won't appeal to everyone – if it is too far out of your comfort zone, don't do it. If you do decide to
go down this route you may wish to receive some professional training. Once
you have built up a reputation it can also provide another source of income.

Where to speak
- Trade associations
- Special interest groups
- Professional associations
- Business groups

What to speak about
Make the title of your talk something that reaches out to people – for example,
'How to Improve Your Confidence by Improving Your Smile'.

Make sure you introduce a system by which those at your talks can contact you, be added to your database and subscribe to your newsletter.

Step 4: Develop strategic alliances

A strategic alliance (SA) is a relationship through which somebody allows you to tell the people in their reservoir what you do, and to invite those people to join your reservoir if they so wish. It also allows your SA partner to tell the people in your reservoir what they do, and invite the people in your reservoir to join theirs. An ideal situation would be where you have a SA with someone who has a reservoir 10 times larger than yours. What is in it for them? A SA partner will look good for having introduced his reservoir to someone who can help them. It is a classic win-win situation.

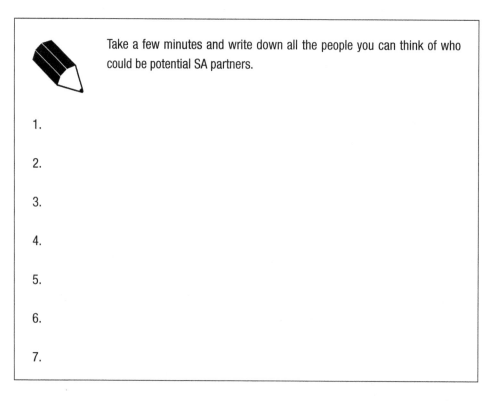

Take a few minutes and write down all the people you can think of who could be potential SA partners.

1.

2.

3.

4.

5.

6.

7.

Step 5: Develop a coordinated internet/social media presence

Since the first edition of this book was published 10 years ago, the landscape has changed enormously as far as using the internet and related media to market you practice. At that time it was just about your website, but today this is just one of a number of possible mechanisms by which you attract people into your virtual reservoir. As Mark Oborn[1] explains:

In conventional marketing you rely on reaching the right person at the right time in the hope that they have the specific problem you are talking about. However, in online marketing the person already knows that they have a problem and is actively searching for a solution. All you have to do is be involved in that search and to stand out.

Your website is still the cornerstone of your online presence and you must optimise it to make sure you get found in those searches described by Mark Oborn. In essence, it is your electronic flypaper for potential future clients. While it is of course entirely possible to use a generic website design, we feel that you get what you pay for and given that this is such an important marketing tool these days you really do need to invest not only money but also time and thought into creating something that stands out from the crowd. Once people reach your site you have to find ways to engage them. You may consider, for example, writing a blog. In his excellent book *Brush*, James Goolnick[2] offers some wise words in this regard:

- Make it fun, otherwise why bother.
- Make the headlines sticky. People have a short attention span, so grab them fast, and then give them something valuable that will make them want to stay.
- Update it regularly, once a week.
- Respect copyright. If you are going to reproduce someone else's work, ask their permission first and quote the source.
- Use multimedia – photographs, links to videos and other relevant sites.
- Take part in the conversation. Remember, if you allow comments you are responsible for all the material that is published on your blog.

Similar advice could be given in relation to other forms of social media (Facebook, Twitter, YouTube, etc.) which, as with blogs, should ideally help patients understand and maintain their dental health in between appointments by providing useful, free, relevant advice. Many dentists are extremely wary of such social media and are reluctant to committing to it. One commonly expressed concern is the risk of adverse comments being posted that deter rather than attract new custom. There are several ways to deal with this and, as always, if you are unsure about how something works, get advice. Just as with blogs, maybe you simply have to engage in the conversation – the worst thing you can do is set up a Facebook page and then never attend it.

REFERENCES

1. www.markoborn.com
2. Goolnick J. *Brush: Proven strategies to make you and your dental business shine.* London: Bow Lane; 2011.

FURTHER READING

- Edwards P, Edwards S. *Teaming Up.* Los Angeles: JP Tarcher; 1997.
- Edwards P, Edwards S. *Getting Business to Come to You.* Los Angeles: JP Tarcher; 1998.
- Misner I. *The World's Best Known Marketing Secret.* Austin, TX: Bard Press; 1994.

CHAPTER NINE

Strategy 8: Maintain a balance between work, rest and play

Work and play are words used to describe the same things under differing conditions.

Mark Twain

Ah, if it were only so simple, but we must strive to find true balance in our lives. This final strategy is more an outcome than a strategy. It is the end result of implementing the first seven strategies.

There are seven key areas of life.

1. *Financial*: all financial matters, both personal and professional.
2. *Business*: all matters to do with your business.
3. *Family*: interactions with nearest and dearest.
4. *Social*: interactions with those outside work and family.
5. *Intellectual*: exercise of the mind on matters outside business.
6. *Physical*: exercise and maintenance of the body.
7. *Spiritual*: expression of heart and soul, rather than the mind.

It is through balancing these diverse aspects of our lives that we can find happiness. When we are out of balance we lose perspective on life, and this can lead to stress, relationships breaking down and work problems appearing unmanageable. In his book *The Secrets of Happiness*, Ben Renshaw[1] observes that one of the quickest routes to unhappiness is comparing ourselves (in all of these respects) with others, and yet we all tend to do it. It is a social condition and we have learnt to do it as a way of measuring our worth:

The truth is you'll come out feeling better about yourself or worse. You'll see yourself as more talented, more attractive and more successful, or the opposite. Either way this isn't going to give you real happiness; it's a temporary fix. Learn to value your uniqueness. Your willingness to give up comparison will enable you to move forwards based on your truth.

BALANCE

Do you have a balanced approach to life? How much time would you ideally like to spend in each of these seven areas?

- Take a typical seven-day week – how much of your waking time is currently spent in each area? (Business owners typically spend 70% of their time on finance and business, 20% on family and 10% spread across the remaining four.)
- If you could wave a realistic magic wand, how would you like to be able to reorganise your time across these seven areas three years from now?
- How about in 10 years?

	Currently	3 years from now	10 years from now
Financial			
Business			
Family			
Social			
Intellectual			
Physical			
Spiritual			

OVERVIEW

If we can summarise how we think you can get to this happy state of balancing work, rest and play, we need to look back over the previous seven strategies.

Vision (*see* Strategy 1)

One of the characteristics of successful people is that they have their three-year vision in place. Have you done yours? If not, go back to Strategy 1 and do it now.

Planning (*see* Strategy 2)

One of the characteristics of successful people is that they take time out to plan and review their lives. If you have not organised your time into free, focus and buffer days and planned time out for personal planning and reflection, go back to Strategy 2 and do it now.

Reserves (*see* Strategy 3)

One of the characteristics of successful people is that they have reserves. Have you created a life in which you have *much* more than you need of the following?

- Time
- Energy
- Space
- Money
- Love
- Skills
- Support
- Nourishing relationships

If not, what needs to happen for you to make significant progress in this area?

Tolerations (*see* Strategy 1)

- What are you putting up with?
- What is draining your energy?
- What do you have to do to eliminate those things that you are tolerating?

Write down your 'top 10 list' of all the things you'd like to have an *absence of* in the next 90 days:

1.   6.

2.   7.

3.   8.

4.   9.

5.   10.

HEALTH AND FITNESS

This goes a long way to improving self-confidence, balance and, ultimately, business performance.

- *Nutrition*: eat and drink sensibly, use your common sense.
- *Sleep*: make sure you have enough sleep.
- *Exercise*: 20 minutes of aerobic exercise three times a week is a great way to keep fit. Something is better than nothing.
- *Meditation*: this can be anything that works for you (running, relaxing in the bath, gazing out of the window even – anything that helps you relax and untangle your thoughts).

What do you need to do to improve in these areas?

As a final thought, consider these three key questions posed by Brian Tracy, one of the world's leading sales trainers:*

- If you had only 10 minutes to live, who would you call and what would you say?

---

* Tracey B. Personal communication.

- If you had only 12 months to live, how would you choose to live it?
- If you could do one truly great thing, what would it be?

Perhaps the best advice we can give as we come to the end of our journey can be found in the words of the anonymous philosopher who wrote:

> *Work like you don't need the money, dance like no one is watching and love like you've never been hurt.*

REFERENCE

1. Renshaw B. *The Secrets of Happiness*. London: Vermilion; 2003.

FURTHER READING

- Alblum M. *Tuesdays with Morrie*. New York: Broadway Books; 2002.
- Bauby JD. *The Diving Bell and the Butterfly*. London: Vintage; 1998.
- Cameron J. *The Artist's Way*. Los Angeles: JP Tarcher; 2002.
- Ferriss T. *The 4-Hour Work Week*. New York: Crown Publishers; 2009.
- Leonard T. *The Portable Coach*. New York: Scribner; 1998.

Self-assessment tools

None will improve your lot
If you yourselves do not.

Bertolt Brecht

One of the most valuable ways to teach yourself new habits is through the vehicle of the self-assessment checklist. In this final section of the book we therefore provide you with five checklist self-assessment tools that apply to all aspects of the eight-strategies programme. These represent a permanent record of the areas in which you can improve and we would actively encourage their use by the whole team to facilitate project management.

- *The Clean Sweep Program*
- *The Dedicated Dentist 100*
- *The Environmental 100*
- *The Financial Control 100*
- *The Customer Journey 100*

There is a small amount of overlap between these tools but that only reflects the degree to which these various aspects of your life interrelate with one another to make you the person you are and to define the life you live.

THE CLEAN SWEEP PROGRAM*

You have more natural energy when you are complete with your physical environment, well-being, money and relationships.

*The Clean Sweep Program** consists of 100 items which, when completed,

---

* *The Clean Sweep Program* was developed by Thomas J Leonard for Coach University.

give you the vitality and strength you want. The programme can be completed in less than one year.

There are four steps to completing the programme:

1. *Answer each question.* If true, tick the appropriate box. Be rigorous; be a hard grader. Only tick the box if the statement is virtually always true for you – if it is only sometimes or usually true, it doesn't count. If the statement doesn't apply to you, so therefore will never be true, then tick the box (you get credit for it, as it will never happen). You may alter statements slightly to more appropriately fit your situation; however, this *must not* be used as a get-out clause to make it easier to score.

2. *Summarise each section.* Add the number of ticks for all four sections and write the amounts where indicated. Then add all four sections together and write your current total along with the date, in the boxes on the right-hand side of the progress chart.

3. *Colour in the progress chart.* If you have nine 'trues' in the well-being section, then colour in the bottom nine boxes, and so on. Always start from the bottom up. The goal is to have the entire chart filled in. In the meantime you will have a current picture of how you are doing in each of the four areas.

4. *Keep playing until all boxes are filled.* You can do it! The process may take 30 days or 360 days, but you **can** achieve a clean sweep! Use your coach or a friend to help you, and once you've achieved it, check back once a year for maintenance.

PROGRESS CHART

Total score

	Environment	Well-being	Money	Relationships	Date	No.
25						
24						
23						
22						
21						
20						
19						
18						
17						
16						
15						
14						
13						
12						
11						
10						
9						
8						
7						
6						
5						
4						
3						
2						
1						

Benefits

In the table provided here, jot down specific benefits, results and breakthroughs that happen in your life because you handled an item on *The Clean Sweep Program*.

Date	Benefit
————	————————————————————————
————	————————————————————————
————	————————————————————————
————	————————————————————————
————	————————————————————————
————	————————————————————————
————	————————————————————————
————	————————————————————————

Physical environment

☐ **Number of ticks**

☐ My personal files, papers and receipts are neatly filed away.

☐ My car is in excellent condition (doesn't need mechanical work, repairs, cleaning or replacing).

☐ My home is clean and tidy (vacuumed, wardrobes and drawers organised, desks and tables clear, furniture in good repair, windows clean).

☐ My appliances, machinery and equipment work well (fridge, toaster, lawnmower, water heater, hi-fi, etc.).

☐ My clothes are all ironed, clean and make me look good (no creases, no piles of washing and no torn, out-of-date or ill-fitting clothes).

☐ My plants and animals are healthy (fed, watered, getting light and love).

☐ My bed/bedroom lets me have the best sleep possible (firm bed, light, air).

☐ I live in a house/flat that I love.

☐ I surround myself with beautiful things.

☐ I live in the geographic location of my choice.

☐ There is ample and healthy lighting around me.

☐ I consistently have adequate time, space and freedom in my life.

☐ Nothing in my environment harms me.

☐ I am not tolerating anything about my home or work environment.

☐ My work environment is productive and inspiring (synergistic, ample tools, no undue pressure).

☐ I recycle.

☐ I use non-ozone-depleting products.

☐ My hair is the way I want it.

☐ I surround myself with music, which makes life more enjoyable.

☐ My bed is made daily.

☐ I don't injure myself, fall or bump into things.

☐ People feel comfortable in my home.

☐ I drink at least two litres of water a day.

☐ I have nothing around the house or in storage that I do not need.

☐ I am consistently early or easily on time.

Well-being

☐ **Number of ticks**

☐ I rarely use caffeine (chocolate, coffee, cola, tea); fewer than three times a week in total.

☐ I rarely eat sugar (fewer than three times a week).

☐ I rarely watch television (fewer than five times a week).

☐ I rarely drink alcohol (fewer than two times a week).

☐ My teeth and gums are healthy (I have seen my dentist in the last six months).

☐ My cholesterol count is healthy.

☐ My blood pressure is healthy.

☐ I have had a complete physical examination in the past three years.

☐ I do not smoke tobacco or other substances.

☐ I do not use illegal drugs or misuse prescribed medications.

☐ I have had a complete eye exam within the past two years (glaucoma check, vision test, etc.).

☐ My weight is within my ideal range.

☐ My nails are healthy and look good.

☐ I don't rush or use adrenaline to get the job done.

☐ I have a rewarding life beyond my work or profession.

☐ I have something to look forward to virtually every day.

☐ I have no habits that I find to be unacceptable to me.

☐ I am aware of the physical or emotional problems or conditions I have, and I am now fully taking care of all of them.

☐ I consistently take weekends and holidays off and take at least four weeks of holiday each year.

☐ I have just the right amount of sleep.

☐ I use well-made sunglasses.

☐ I do not suffer.

☐ I laugh out loud every day.

☐ I walk or exercise at least three times a week.

☐ I hear well.

Money

❐ I currently save at least 10% of my income.

❐ I pay my bills on time.

❐ My income source/revenue base is stable and predictable.

❐ I know how much I must have to be financially independent and I have a plan to get there.

❐ I have returned and made good on any money borrowed.

❐ I have written agreements and am current with payments to individuals or companies to whom I owe money.

❐ I have six months of living expenses in an easily accessible account.

❐ I live on a weekly budget, which allows me to save and not suffer.

❐ All my tax returns have been filed and all my taxes have been paid.

❐ I currently live well, within my means.

❐ I have excellent personal insurance (life, accident disability, medical, etc.).

❐ My assets (car, home, possessions and treasures) are well insured.

❐ I have a financial plan for the next year.

❐ I have no legal clouds hanging over me.

❐ My will is up to date and accurate.

❐ Any parking tickets, alimony or child support are paid and current.

❐ My investments do not keep me awake at night.

❐ I know how much I am worth.

❐ I am on a career, professional, business track that is or will soon be financially and personally rewarding.

❐ My earnings are commensurate with the effort I put into my job.

❐ I have no 'loose ends' at work.

❐ I am in a relationship with people who can assist in my career/professional development.

❐ I rarely miss work because of illness.

❐ I am putting aside enough money each month to reach financial independence.

❐ My earnings outpace inflation, consistently.

Relationships

❐ **Number of ticks**

❐ I have told my parents in the last three months that I love them.

❐ I get along well with my sibling(s).

❐ I get along well with my co-workers/clients.

❐ I get along well with my manager/staff.

❐ There is no one I would dread or feel uncomfortable 'running across' (in the street, at the airport, at a party).

❐ I put people first and results second.

❐ I have let go of the relationships that drag me down or damage me ('let go' means to end, walk away from, declare complete, no longer be attached to).

❐ I have communicated or attempted to communicate with everyone whom I have damaged, injured or seriously upset, even if it wasn't my fault.

❐ I do not gossip or talk about others.

❐ I have a circle of friends/family who love me for who I am more than just what I do for them.

❐ I tell people how they can satisfy me.

❐ I am fully caught up with letters and calls.

❐ I always tell the truth, no matter what.

❐ I receive enough love from those around me to feel good.

❐ I have fully forgiven those people who have hurt or damaged me, intentionally or not.

❐ I am a person of my word. People can count on me.

❐ I quickly correct miscommunications and misunderstandings when they occur.

❐ I live life on my terms, not by the rules or preferences of others.

❐ I am complete with past loves or spouses.

❐ I am in tune with my wants/needs and get them taken care of.

❐ I do not judge or criticise others.

❐ I do not 'take personally' the things people say to me.

❐ I have a best friend or a soulmate.

❐ I make requests rather than complain.

❐ I spend time with people who don't try to change me.

Congratulations on completing *The Clean Sweep Program*! Revisit the programme until you get 80+ ticks. Remember, every professional's experience will be different. Be kind to yourself and work at your own pace. There is no one right way to get 80+! Good luck.

THE DEDICATED DENTIST 100*

The Dedicated Dentist 100 is a tool to assess areas of your practice. Use it to identify areas for focus. The intention is to make your practice one of the most progressive within the profession. It focuses on four areas of your practice:
- strong patient relationships
- practice management
- your team of professionals
- personal development and balance.

There are three steps to completing *The Dedicated Dentist 100*:
1. *Answer each question*. If the statement is true, tick the box. If not, leave it blank until you have done what it takes for it to be a full yes. Be rigorous; be a tough marker. Only tick the box if the statement is virtually always true for you – if it is only sometimes or usually true, it doesn't count. However, if the statement doesn't apply to you, so therefore will never be true, then tick the box (you get credit for it, as it will never happen). You may also modify statements slightly to more appropriately fit your situation – but this *must not* be used as a get-out clause to make it easier to score!
2. *Summarise each section*. Add up the number of ticks and note the total at the end of each section. Then transfer the total of each section, along with the date, to the spaces in the '*My progress record*'. As you continue to work the programme, your totals will change. Use this section to track your progress.
3. *Keep playing until all the boxes are filled*. This process may take 30 days or two years, but you can do it! It's not the time that matters, it's that you are moving forward and achieving results.

---

* Philip Cohen and Laura Hess, coaches and partners in SPARCK INTERNATIONAL, created this survey. It is based on concepts found in the Professional Practice Checklist created by Thomas J Leonard and Coach University.

MY PROGRESS RECORD

Date	Strong patient relationships	Practice management	Your team of professionals	Personal development and balance	Make a note here of any specific benefits or breakthroughs as you work the programme
	❏	❏	❏	❏	
	❏	❏	❏	❏	
	❏	❏	❏	❏	
	❏	❏	❏	❏	
	❏	❏	❏	❏	
	❏	❏	❏	❏	

Strong patient relationships

❏ **Number of ticks**

Patients come to a dentist because of his or her reputation or availability. They stay with a dentist because of the service they receive and because of the relationship that both parties create. Patients expect you to be a highly skilled communicator.

❏ I listen to and hear what my patients want.

❏ I anticipate patients' concerns before they voice them.

❏ I fully involve patients in treatment planning. I explain options and consequences.

❏ I respond directly to questions asked by patients.

❏ We speak clearly, simply and without jargon when offering recommendations or answering patients' questions.

❏ My receptionist warmly welcomes each caller and patient to my practice.

❏ I am unconditionally constructive when I speak.

❏ Team members participate in communication skills training.

❏ A patient is more than a customer. We treat patients with concern and respect.

❏ We show interest in our patients by remembering things of interest to them.

❏ We regard and treat our patients as consumers who have a choice in who provides their dental care.

☐ There is complete trust between us and our patients. They tell us everything we need to know to serve them professionally.

☐ We use conversations and surveys to involve patients in our continual improvement.

☐ We manage our time and our patients' time well – waiting is virtually non-existent.

☐ Patients view our service as valuable, safe and friendly. Our patients leave the practice feeling they have received the very best service available anywhere.

☐ We inform our patients how to maintain and improve the supply of information to us.

☐ Our patients know we want (and expect) their honest feedback about every part of our practice.

☐ Team members have completely resolved all situations in which patients were dissatisfied with our services or us.

☐ Our patients understand and believe that quality consistency and delivery is our primary concern.

☐ Our objective is to establish and maintain lifetime relationships with our patients.

☐ We don't gossip or make disparaging statements about our patients.

☐ We send out a regular newsletter or announcement to patients.

☐ Patients aren't alone for long periods in the practice.

☐ We don't discuss one patient in front of another.

☐ Our phones are answered professionally. Callers don't wait on hold and neither are they likely to get an answerphone, except after hours.

Practice management

☐ **Number of ticks**

How you operate your practice affects your effectiveness, profitability and enjoyment. Every practice has hidden costs – emotional costs – which limit the quality of service provided and keep the practice less than full.

☐ I quickly refer out patients whom I cannot help easily or who bring out my worst side.

☐ Our patients keep their appointments.

☐ We are experts at presenting the treatment plan.

☐ We have a programme to reactivate past patients.

☐ We receive ___% of our patients via referral.

❐ We maintain strong relationships with at least six centres of influence who send lots of referrals.

❐ Our patients know all the services we offer and the type of patients we are looking for.

❐ We call or thank the source of every referral.

❐ We make it easy for new patients to contact us.

❐ We have written material, such as a card or brochure, for our patients to give others.

❐ Our practice's goals and objectives emphasise attracting, scheduling and completing the maximum production each day through teamwork.

❐ We have learnt how to make a profit on all work performed.

❐ Mistakes are handled immediately and without judgement or consequences.

❐ Our practice is clean, neat and well kept. It represents us well.

❐ Our practice is well equipped. Each surgery stands alone and is set up with the finest instruments.

❐ We have the right accountant, banker, solicitor, coach and other advisers, all whom add to our profitability.

❐ We have a multifaceted welcome pack that we offer to patients regularly. This includes short-, intermediate- and long-term goals, along with a mission statement for the practice.

❐ The practice is in good enough shape to sell.

❐ Bank reconciliations are complete and up to date.

❐ All income, sales, property and payroll taxes are current.

❐ All bills are paid on time.

❐ The accounting department is well run and/or we use a superb bookkeeping service and/or auditor. Monthly financial statements are prepared and reviewed by the fifteenth of each month.

❐ Accounts receivable tracking is in place. We collect at least 95% of all fees.

❐ The practice is as profitable as, or more so than, others in the same geographical area.

❐ The practice has a practice manual that fully explains all practice procedures and protocols.

Your team of professionals

☐ **Number of ticks**

Team members need encouragement to be their best. They also need direction and freedom to do their jobs. Providing a supportive environment for your team's personal and professional development increases loyalty, improves morale and enhances their involvement in your practice's success.

☐ Team members have warm, comforting and sensitive phone, reception and chair-side styles. We provide training in these skills to all team members.

☐ Everyone knows and understands the value of our services and purpose of our practice.

☐ Each team member knows the meaning of value-added service.

☐ We rely on user-friendly systems and checklists to monitor our performance.

☐ Our patients are compassionately informed when they violate any of our personal or professional boundaries.

☐ We work hard without suffering or bringing imbalance to our personal/ emotional life.

☐ We don't complain or blame. Rather, we make requests, offer solutions and clarify patient resistance.

☐ We have a supportive coach or mentor available to help us maintain an emotionally cost-free practice.

☐ We hire people with the best work ethic and team spirit.

☐ Team members are absolutely clear on their roles and responsibilities.

☐ Each member of the team is responsible for the day-to-day decisions affecting his or her goals, objectives and areas of responsibility.

☐ Everyone operates as a team member with open communication at all times.

☐ I recognise coaching, training and education are required to allow my team to achieve its full potential.

☐ My team is excellent! They are skilled, motivated and integrated. I am proud to have them represent me.

☐ Team members are required to take continuing education programmes.

☐ Team members are responsible for getting their jobs done and their needs met.

☐ There is mutual respect between team members.

☐ Communication skills are taught and practised by team members.

☐ Team members are well paid, including benefits and profit share.

☐ Team meetings are productive and meaningful. All team members attend.

☐ Quarterly reviews are conducted with each team member.
☐ Team members look for ways to increase production and revenue and to improve the practice.
☐ At least once a year we have a consultant or coach observe our practice.
☐ Team members support each other by filling in when needed.
☐ Our practice is a place of preferred employment.

Personal development and balance

☐ **Number of ticks**

The quality of the dentist's work and the success of the practice depends heavily on how high the dentist maintains his or her well-being physically, emotionally, mentally and spiritually.

☐ I speak the truth as I see it. I don't withhold, lie or exaggerate.
☐ I delegate daily office responsibilities to my practice manager, so I can focus on delivering excellent dentistry.
☐ My technical excellence is reinforced through monthly seminars, continuing education and/or study groups.
☐ I have a plan in case I become disabled or die.
☐ I spend quality time with my family and we enjoy one another very much.
☐ I am able to maintain a fresh perspective, innovate, learn and improve, because I have enough time and everything is so well done or delegated.
☐ I have a gifted right-hand person/executive assistant who handles every business and personal detail. I don't get distracted or diverted.
☐ I have a strong, happy and healthy personal life, with lots of physical activity and pleasure. Work is work and not my life.
☐ I am adrenaline free: I am not driven.
☐ I put aside plenty of money so I can be financially independent early.
☐ I have the property, liability, life and disability insurance appropriate for me. All policies are reviewed annually.
☐ I have a plan for my retirement and sale of my practice.
☐ I know my net worth.
☐ My personal relationships are healthy and happy.
☐ There is no one in my life I want to avoid or I dread spending time with.
☐ I have fun outside work every day.
☐ My commute to work is enjoyable.
☐ My practice is fulfilling and satisfying.
☐ I walk or exercise at least three times a week.

☐ I am not tolerating anything in my work environment.

☐ I make full use of my holiday time, pursuing non-work-related activities.

☐ I live within my current financial means. I don't worry about money.

☐ My will is up to date.

☐ I have a circle of friends and family who appreciate me for who I am, not for what I do.

☐ I am a person of my word. People can count on me.

Congratulations on completing *The Dedicated Dentist 100*! Revisit the programme until you get 80+ ticks. Remember, every professional's experience will be different. Be kind to yourself and work at your own pace. There is no one right way to get 80+! Good luck.

THE ENVIRONMENTAL 100*

The Environmental 100 is a tool to assess the environmental health of your business. Use it to identify areas for focus. The intention is to help you become well organised and to create a more pleasant working environment. (You may also learn yours is already among the best!) It focuses on five areas:

- sight
- sound
- touch
- smell/taste
- relationships/culture.

There are three steps to completing *The Environmental 100*:

1. *Answer each question.* If the statement is true, tick the box. If not, leave it blank until you have done what it takes for it to be a full yes. Be rigorous; be a tough marker. Only tick the box if the statement is virtually always true for you – if it is only sometimes or usually true, it doesn't count. However, if the statement doesn't apply to you, so therefore will never be true, then tick the box (you get credit for it, as it will never happen). You may also modify statements slightly to more appropriately fit your situation – but this *must not* be used as a get-out clause to make it easier to score!

2. *Summarise each section.* Add up the number of ticks and note the total at the end of each section. Then transfer the total of each section, along with the date, to the spaces in the '*My progress record*'. As you continue to work the programme, your totals will change. Use this section to track your progress.

---

* Chris Barrow and Julian Cotton of Sapience created *The Environmental 100*. You may make copies of this assessment as long as you use it in its entirety, including reprinting this statement on each page.

3. *Keep playing until all the boxes are filled.* This process may take 30 days or two years, but you can do it! It's not the time that matters, it's that you are moving forward and achieving results.

MY PROGRESS RECORD

Date	Sight	Sound	Touch	Smell/taste	Relationships/culture	Make a note here of any specific benefits or breakthroughs as you work the programme
	❑	❑	❑	❑	❑	
	❑	❑	❑	❑	❑	
	❑	❑	❑	❑	❑	
	❑	❑	❑	❑	❑	
	❑	❑	❑	❑	❑	
	❑	❑	❑	❑	❑	

Sight: How things *look* in our business

❑ **Number of ticks**

❑ My workspace is neat and well organised.
❑ My clothing is clean, comfortable and appropriate.
❑ I have had a complete eye examination within the last two years.
❑ There is sufficient natural light.
❑ I have personalised my own workspace.
❑ The light in my workspace allows me to perform all tasks.
❑ I rarely suffer from headaches at work.
❑ I either do not need corrective lenses or wear lenses as prescribed.
❑ Colours in my workplace are pleasant and stimulating
❑ I either do not use VDU (visual display unit) screens as part of my work or use VDUs and I am allowed regular breaks.
❑ Either I do not use a VDU or my screen is always free from glare and distortion.
❑ My workplace is cleaned on a regular basis.
❑ Space is distributed fairly and evenly.
❑ There are natural plants and flowers.
❑ I never endanger myself or colleagues.

☐ I am happy with my own appearance.
☐ I regularly discard unwanted papers.
☐ I turn off lights when last out of a room.
☐ The bulbs in our lights are energy efficient.
☐ My environment is aesthetically pleasing.

Sound: what you *hear* in our business

☐ **Number of ticks**

☐ There is an absence of excessive noise around my workstation.
☐ There are no disruptive appliances or machines within my workplace.
☐ I hear well.
☐ I do not regularly use a mobile phone.
☐ I do not distract colleagues with my own sounds.
☐ Workplace sounds are pleasant and invigorating.
☐ I have access to quiet areas.
☐ I either do not need assistance to hear well or wear artificial hearing aids as prescribed.
☐ I never shout at colleagues.
☐ I listen carefully to clients and colleagues.
☐ Necessary ear protectors are available or are not required.
☐ I either never need protective ear equipment or utilise appropriate protection as necessary.
☐ Communication is open and effective.
☐ I do not vindictively gossip or talk about others.
☐ There are regular fire alarm tests.
☐ I am familiar with all alarm sounds.
☐ Open praise is commonplace.
☐ The telephone system is up to date.
☐ Conversation is polite and positive.
☐ I am always open to comments and assistance from others.

Touch: how it *feels* in our business

☐ **Number of ticks**

☐ I have sufficient space in which to work.
☐ My environment feels productive and inspiring.
☐ My work environment feels safe and secure.

- ❏ I am not damaged within my workspace.
- ❏ I have nothing in my workspace that I do not need.
- ❏ The temperature at work is always comfortable.
- ❏ The humidity within my workspace is always acceptable.
- ❏ Furniture is appropriate and comfortable.
- ❏ My chair is well maintained.
- ❏ My workplace is arranged efficiently and safely.
- ❏ I feel well rested and replenished when I arrive at work.
- ❏ I am allowed to take regular breaks.
- ❏ I am not tolerating anything bad about my work experience.
- ❏ I feel happy about my weight.
- ❏ I walk or take exercise at least three times a week.
- ❏ My blood pressure is at a healthy level.
- ❏ My cholesterol count is healthy.
- ❏ I have had a complete medical within the last three years.
- ❏ All equipment is fit for its purpose.
- ❏ I take regular breaks.

Smell/taste: the *aromas and nutrition* experienced in our business

❏ **Number of ticks**

- ❏ There are no offensive smells within my work area.
- ❏ There are pleasant, invigorating aromas surrounding me.
- ❏ The aromas of others do not offend me.
- ❏ The air is pure and fresh.
- ❏ My aroma doesn't offend others (smoking/perfume/body odour).
- ❏ I have access to good-quality drinking water at work.
- ❏ I am a non-smoker.
- ❏ I rarely drink alcohol (fewer than 10 units a week).
- ❏ I can obtain a nutritional meal at work.
- ❏ I have access to an appropriate separate food consumption area.
- ❏ I drink plenty of water.
- ❏ I have access to a food preparation area.
- ❏ Toilets are clean and fragrant.
- ❏ There is a positive, healthy atmosphere at work.
- ❏ I eat fresh fruit every day.
- ❏ I consume vegetables regularly.
- ❏ I avoid snacking on sweets and crisps.
- ❏ I always eat breakfast.

☐ My teeth and gums are healthy.
☐ I rarely consume caffeine (chocolate, tea, coffee, cola, etc.).

Relationships/culture: the *health* of our business

☐ **Number of ticks**

☐ There is a supportive and positive culture throughout the company.
☐ I have a healthy balance between home and work.
☐ I have a healthy relationship with all my colleagues.
☐ I have a good relationship with my manager.
☐ I put people first and results second.
☐ The business puts people first and results second.
☐ I am up to date with all letters and calls.
☐ I am worthy of trust; people can depend upon me.
☐ There is a culture of openness and trust within the business.
☐ I either prevent or resolve conflict.
☐ I am always willing to help/coach others.
☐ Innovation is encouraged and rewarded.
☐ The rewards of success are shared.
☐ All individuals are treated with equal value.
☐ People understand what is expected of them.
☐ Leaders in the business set a good example.
☐ Safety is a priority in our business.
☐ I enjoy my work.
☐ I am consistently early or on time.
☐ Staff receive regular and appropriate training.

Congratulations on completing *The Environmental 100*! Revisit the programme until you get 80+ ticks. Remember every professional's experience will be different. Be kind to yourself and work at your own pace to 80+! Good luck.

THE FINANCIAL CONTROL 100*

The Financial Control 100 is a tool to assess your level of financial organisation. Use it to identify areas for focus. The intention is to help you become financially well organised and to create a plan that will make you bulletproof. It focuses on four areas of your finances:

- personal finances
- borrowing and saving
- financial planning
- business finance.

There are three steps to completing *The Financial Control 100*:

1. *Answer each question.* If the statement is true, tick the box. If not, leave it blank until you have done what it takes for it to be a full yes. Be rigorous; be a tough marker. Only tick the box if the statement is virtually always true for you – if it is only sometimes or usually true, it doesn't count. However, if the statement doesn't apply to you, so therefore will never be true, then tick the box (you get credit for it, as it will never happen). You may also modify statements slightly to more appropriately fit your situation – but this *must not* be used as a get-out clause to make it easier to score!

2. *Summarise each section.* Add up the number of ticks and note the total at the end of each section. Then transfer the total of each section, along with the date, to the spaces in the '*My progress record*'. As you continue to work the programme, your totals will change. Use this section to track your progress.

3. *Keep playing until all the boxes are filled.* This process may take 30 days or two years, but you can do it! It's not the time that matters, it's that you are moving forward and achieving results.

---

* Chris Barrow of The Business Coaching Co. Ltd created *The Financial Control 100*. You may make copies of this assessment as long as you use it in its entirety, including reprinting this statement on each page.

MY PROGRESS RECORD

Date	Personal finances	Borrowing and saving	Financial planning	Business finance	Make a note here of any specific benefits or breakthroughs as you work the programme
	❒	❒	❒	❒	
	❒	❒	❒	❒	
	❒	❒	❒	❒	
	❒	❒	❒	❒	
	❒	❒	❒	❒	
	❒	❒	❒	❒	

Personal finances

❒ **Number of ticks**

❒ I have prepared a personal financial budget for the current calendar year.

❒ I review my personal budget on a monthly basis and always look for opportunities to cut costs.

❒ I know what my regular income is.

❒ Once a year I review the premiums that I pay for building, contents and motor insurance.

❒ I pay my credit card bills on time to avoid unnecessary interest charges.

❒ I reduce the cost of my utility bills by payment on direct debit mandate.

❒ I constantly review the cost of charge cards and credit cards to make sure I am using the most competitive facilities.

❒ I have a personal filing system for my finances, which is kept neat, orderly and up to date.

❒ Once a year I review the deal I am getting from my bankers and look around for a better package.

❒ I never use another bank's cash dispenser to withdraw cash, in view of the excess charges that they may impose.

❒ I constantly review my expenditure on energy and look at ways of reducing my home heating bills.

❒ Once a year I review my utility providers to make sure that I am getting the best deal possible.

❒ I never accept a utility bill that is based upon an estimate of consumption – I always 'read the meter'.

❏ Once a year I review my telephone provider and look at ways of reducing my call costs by switching service or using a discount scheme.

❏ All of my personal chattels are insured for their full replacement value.

❏ My home is fully secured with locking windows, doors and a burglar alarm system so that I can obtain a discount for my home insurance.

❏ My no claims bonus is insured on my motor insurance policy.

❏ Whenever I am granted air miles or reward points I make sure I use them.

❏ I have created resources of cash to deal with emergencies and opportunities.

❏ I meet with my bank manager annually to review our relationship.

❏ Once every five years I check my credit rating.

❏ I keep an updated list of the contents of my home and their value.

❏ All of my personal bank reconciliations are up to date.

❏ When I buy something, I buy the best possible quality.

❏ I always pay my bills on time.

Borrowing and saving

❏ **Number of ticks**

❏ I have returned or made good on any short-term money I borrowed from individuals.

❏ I have written agreements and I am up to date with payments to individuals or companies to whom I owe money personally.

❏ I have no legal clouds hanging over me.

❏ I never, ever go over my borrowing limits.

❏ I have converted any hard-core overdraft to medium-term loan and reduced the servicing costs.

❏ I review my mortgage once a year to make sure that I am getting the best deal and have looked at flexible mortgages and drawdown facilities.

❏ I don't borrow more than 90% of the value of my property to avoid paying any mortgage indemnity insurance.

❏ I occasionally use my property mortgages to consolidate long-term debt.

❏ I have selected the correct repayment method for my property-secured loans.

❏ Once a year I review the annual percentage rate of my short- and long-term borrowing to make sure that I am getting the best deal.

❏ I have ensured that all mortgages/loans and/or overdrafts are self-cancelling, or can be serviced in the event of my death, disability or critical illness.

☐ I regularly transfer surplus cash from current account to an interest-bearing savings account.

☐ I keep a three-month reserve of personal running expenses at all times.

☐ I save small amounts on a regular basis.

☐ I understand my own attitude to risk and know how much I want to invest in guaranteed investments and asset-backed investments.

☐ I use all of my tax-free savings allowances.

☐ I maximise my pension allowances.

☐ I make sure that any savings products that I buy are fully portable, should my circumstances change.

☐ I put away plenty of funds with which to become financially independent early.

☐ I have ensured that my capital is invested, as it should be, to protect it from inflation and to maintain my lifestyle both now and in the future.

☐ I have reduced, where possible, the tax I pay on my capital investments.

☐ Once a year I review the family's wills to ensure that my estate will pass to the beneficiaries of my choice rather than to the Inland Revenue.

☐ I set personal financial goals for three months hence, one year hence, and three years hence.

☐ I use the services of an independent financial adviser.

☐ I am sure that my tax coding is correct.

Financial planning

☐ **Number of ticks**

☐ All my tax returns are filed on time to avoid penalties and interest.

☐ All my taxes are paid on time to avoid penalties and interest.

☐ I have sent a form BR19 to the Department for Work and Pensions to check my state pension entitlement.

☐ I have created a financial plan, which gives me a clear grasp of my present financial situation and helps me to make the most effective use of my resources towards the achievement of my goals and objectives.

☐ I have ensured that, in the event of my death, my spouse/family would inherit my home, free of mortgage, and have sufficient capital/income to maintain their normal standard of living.

☐ I have ensured that in the event of my spouse's death, I would have sufficient capital/income to maintain my normal standard of living and to fund some additional help in the home.

☐ I have ensured that in the event of my illness, including a critical illness such as heart attack, cancer or stroke, that my family and I would have sufficient capital/income to maintain our normal standard of living.

☐ I am planning to create a lifelong inflation-resistant pension payable from my desired age.

☐ I am planning to create a lifelong inflation-resistant pension for my spouse.

☐ I am providing for the cost of educating my children or grandchildren and ensuring that this would remain possible in the event of my death, disability or critical illness.

☐ I have a plan to achieve financial independence.

☐ In the event of my needing long-term nursing care, I have ensured that the costs can be met so that my home and other assets will pass to my family and not to the state.

☐ I have taken steps to reduce my family's potential inheritance tax liability and ensure that sufficient cash will be available, in the right hands at the right time, to meet any remaining liability.

☐ I have considered the use of offshore banking, investments, trusts and trading companies, to improve the performance and tax effectiveness of my personal and business assets, without any increase in risk.

☐ I have identified the most tax-efficient method of taking remuneration from my business.

☐ I have identified suitable tax strategies that may reduce or eliminate unnecessary taxation.

☐ I have no financial stress of any kind in my life.

☐ I have a team of professional advisers around me who are able to help me in maintaining my financial plan.

☐ My income source and revenue base is stable and predictable.

☐ My earnings are commensurate with the effort I put into my job.

☐ I have no 'loose ends' at work.

☐ My earnings outpace inflation consistently.

☐ I've set up my business to be more profit driven than growth driven.

☐ I am naturally cautious about spending money although I am willing to invest cash in my business to make even more profit.

☐ My target market is well defined, they can afford to buy my product and services, and I can access my target market easily with the contacts and tools that I have.

Business finance

❑ **Number of ticks**

❑ I pay cash even for capital expenditures.

❑ There is a strong, profitable future in my field.

❑ There is not much financial risk to me the way I have set up my business. I can afford the mistakes that will be made.

❑ I am not over-borrowing and I am not pushing to maximise every single opportunity. I have patience for the market to decide and buy.

❑ I have future plans for additional products and revenue streams.

❑ I know what my gross profit margins are.

❑ I know what my net profit needs to be to support my desired lifestyle.

❑ I know my cash flow needs.

❑ I know my daily/weekly/monthly/yearly sales goals and results.

❑ I know how quickly I collect my debts.

❑ I know my referral rate as a percentage of my sales.

❑ I know my current and aged debtors and creditors.

❑ Bank reconciliations for the business are complete and up to date.

❑ All income, sales and property taxes are paid up to date.

❑ We have learnt how to make a profit on all the work we perform.

❑ All bills are paid on time.

❑ The internal accounting function is well run and/or we use a superb bookkeeping service and/or accountant.

❑ We have budgets, which we compare with our monthly financial statements by the tenth of each month.

❑ My business profits are 20% more than that of other similar businesses in the same geographical area.

❑ We collect our debts within 90 days.

❑ Our services and products are packaged so that they produce a stream of income, not just a one-time sale.

❑ We produce monthly management accounts and analyse them on a monthly basis.

❑ I know that my prices are right.

❑ We have three months' emergency funds in the business.

❑ We have properly planned and financed capital projects in the business over the next three years.

Congratulations on completing *The Financial 100*! Remember, every professional's experience will be different. Be kind to yourself and work at your own pace. There is no one right way to get 80+! Good luck.

THE CUSTOMER JOURNEY 100*

The Customer Journey 100 is a tool to assess the customer service experience in your business. Use it to identify areas for focus. The intention is to make your practice one of the most progressive within your sector. It focuses on six areas:

- foundations for success
- the patient journey I
- the patient journey II
- ethical selling skills
- the patient journey III
- the welcome pack.

There are three steps to completing *The Customer Journey 100*:

1. *Answer each question.* If the statement is true, tick the box. If not, leave it blank until you have done what it takes for it to be a full yes. Be rigorous; be a tough marker. Only tick the box if the statement is virtually always true for you – if it is only sometimes or usually true, it doesn't count. However, if the statement doesn't apply to you, so therefore will never be true, then tick the box (you get credit for it, as it will never happen). You may also modify statements slightly to more appropriately fit your situation – but this *must not* be used as a get-out clause to make it easier to score!
2. *Summarise each section.* Add up the number of ticks and note the total at the end of each section. Then transfer the total of each section, along with the date, to the spaces in the '*My progress record*'. As you continue to work the programme, your totals will change. Use this section to track your progress.
3. *Keep playing until all the boxes are filled.* This process may take 30 days or two years, but you can do it! It's not the time that matters, it's that you are moving forward and achieving results.

---

* Chris Barrow created *The Customer Journey 100*. Special thanks to Ashley Latter of www.thesellingcoach. com for his contribution to the 'Ethical selling skills' section.

MY PROGRESS RECORD

Date	Foundations for success	The patient journey I	The patient journey II	Ethical selling skills	The patient journey III	The welcome pack	Make a note here of any specific benefits or breakthroughs as you work the programme
	❐	❐	❐	❐	❐	❐	
	❐	❐	❐	❐	❐	❐	
	❐	❐	❐	❐	❐	❐	
	❐	❐	❐	❐	❐	❐	
	❐	❐	❐	❐	❐	❐	
	❐	❐	❐	❐	❐	❐	

Foundations for success

❐ **Number of ticks**

It has been said that you cannot make progress as an individual or with a team from a start point of low self-esteem. In this section we explore the potential market and the attitudes that will be necessary for your prosperity.

❐ We have created sufficient time in the appointment book to enable us to deliver our ideal service.

❐ We follow a programme of continuous professional education to ensure our ability to deliver our products/services with excellence.

❐ We follow a programme of continuous development in customer service.

❐ We follow a programme of continuous development in ethical selling skills.

❐ We allow brainstorm rules when discussing new ideas.

❐ We understand the implication of demographics and economics in recognising our ideal clients.

❐ We recognise the future economic potential of the market we are serving.

❐ We appreciate that our products/services will be in demand – the question is 'who will the customer buy them from?'

❐ We understand the quality/price/time triangle and have chosen high-quality products/services and customer service, along with convenient timing/environment as our focus.

❐ We do not compromise on our prices.

❐ We all feel that we are paid adequately for what we do.

☐ An element of our pay is related to the performance of the whole business.

☐ We feel appreciated by our employer.

☐ We appreciate one another.

☐ We appreciate the customers who we serve.

☐ We are appreciated by our customers.

☐ We have fun at work.

☐ We enjoy the physical environment in which we work.

☐ We have high self-esteem as individuals. We are '10 out of 10s'.

☐ We have high self-esteem as a team. We are '10 out of 10s'.

☐ We understand that life is a series of 'mountains, valleys and missiles' and do not allow that to affect our '10'.

☐ We have a 'helium culture' in our business – when we communicate, we do so in a way that increases the listener's self-esteem.

☐ We are professional actors at work – we do not have 'bad hair days'.

☐ We understand that our customers pass through the business like batons in a relay race – and that part of our job is to prevent the baton from dropping.

☐ We understand that a 'WOW' customer journey consists of structure (the physical environment), process (how the customer is dealt with as an individual) and outcome (does the customer receive his or her desired outcome?).

☐ We recognise that selling can be ethical if delivered in the correct way.

☐ We recognise that ethical selling is about helping customers to buy the products and services that are suitable and desired.

The patient journey I

☐ **Number of ticks**

Receptionists can be called the 'managing directors of first impressions'. All of the team are involved in meeting and greeting new customers. In this section we explore the creation of those first impressions.

☐ When we answer the phone we smile, greet, introduce ourselves by name and enquire.

☐ When we greet a customer personally, we smile, make eye contact, acknowledge, introduce ourselves by name and enquire.

☐ We always find out how our new clients would like to be addressed so we don't run the risk of alienating them by being too familiar.

☐ When we are questioned about our products and services we do not simply hand over literature. We ask 'what is it about _____ that you are interested in?'

☐ We have permission to use our intuition and respectfully say 'no' to inappropriate customers.

☐ We have developed appropriate language for this.

☐ We always ask customers whether they would like to book an appointment.

☐ We can deal with concerns and objections using the 'feel, felt, found' technique in a genuine way.

☐ We always introduce appropriate special offers into the conversation.

☐ We recognise the opportunity to cross-sell our other products and services.

☐ We understand how to create an 'elevator speech' to explain the benefits of what we do.

☐ We have heard 'elevator speeches' from all of the team.

☐ We understand that 'no' can mean 'no, never' or 'no, not now' and we have a diary system to remind customers when asked.

☐ We understand the concept of a reservoir of future sales.

The patient journey II

☐ **Number of ticks**

From reception to consultation – key skills are needed to deal with delay and to 'pass the baton' carefully.

☐ If customers are late to arrive, we have a system and language to deal with this.

☐ When customers are delayed because we are late, we keep them posted frequently. We have a system and language to deal with this.

☐ We explain that delays occur because we are helping other customers.

☐ We have an appropriate environment in which customers can wait for a meeting/consultation.

☐ When we greet customers on the premises, we make eye contact, smile and introduce ourselves.

☐ We have a system by which customers are escorted through our premises.

Ethical selling skills

☐ **Number of ticks**

Successful business is 98% understanding people and 2% technical knowledge. You must have 100% of the 2% – but it's the 98% that makes the sale.

☐ We begin our relationship with our customers by building rapport. We understand how to do this.

☐ We then move on to review their interests as expressed on our menu.

☐ We understand that a blank menu does not necessarily mean a lack of interest.

☐ We understand the distinction between products/services, features and outcomes. We focus on the customer's desired outcome.

☐ We can and know when to ask 'current situation' questions.

☐ We can and know when to ask 'benefit' questions.

☐ We can and know when to ask 'barrier' questions.

☐ We can and know when to ask 'outcome' questions.

☐ We understand how to construct a capability statement when making recommendations.

☐ We include a description of the factual recommendation.

☐ We bridge this into a benefit statement.

☐ We remind the customer of the outcome.

☐ We offer evidence.

☐ We ask for trial commitment.

☐ We understand how to resolve concerns and objections at this point.

☐ We make a 'cushion' statement.

☐ We reflect and clarify the concern to ensure our understanding.

☐ We identify any hidden objections.

☐ We respond with solutions, explanations, education, options, evidence or value.

☐ We ask for a trial commitment when the concern is resolved.

☐ When challenged on price we request clarification – 'is the concern about value or timing?'

☐ We can offer payment timing options to resolve this concern.

☐ We understand how to gain final commitment.

☐ We can and know when to ask direct commitment questions.

☐ We can and know when to use alternative choices.

☐ We can and know when to use minor points.

☐ We can and know when to request a move to the next step.

☐ We can and know when to utilise future opportunities.

☐ We can and know when to use a weighing method for larger decisions.

☐ We know how to present our recommendations in writing and how to discuss them.

The patient journey III

☐ **Number of ticks**

When the customer has made a successful purchase, the work of building a lifelong relationship begins. Here we examine how to build that lifetime customer and have them introduce their friends and family.

☐ We have a system and language to request testimonial letters.
☐ We keep a testimonial folder on our premises.
☐ We have a referral card.
☐ We have a system and language to distribute referral cards.
☐ We have a system to follow up on testimonial letters.
☐ We have systems and language to request payment.
☐ We give our customers options for payment, so as to accommodate timing – but we don't compromise on price.
☐ We always book our next meeting with customers.
☐ We have an 'end of transaction' letter and a system for its issue.
☐ We know that 'attitude, not aptitude, determines altitude'.

The welcome pack

☐ **Number of ticks**

It's a great idea to establish boundaries at the start of a new relationship – and to expose yourself to the risk of doing business. A well-designed welcome pack will save you time and money.

☐ We have created a welcome pack for our business.
☐ It includes a covering letter outlining the customer's first 'journey'.
☐ It contains a copy of our mission statement.
☐ There is a 'meet the team' section.
☐ It includes necessary directions/parking details.
☐ We include our terms and conditions of business.
☐ There is a 'promises' section.
☐ There is a price guide.
☐ There is a menu of our 'top 10 outcomes'.
☐ The language of the menu is 'outcome' followed by 'feature', followed by product/service description.

❒ We include any preliminary paperwork for the customer to complete and also explain the benefit to the customer of completion.

❒ We appreciate that some prospective customers will cancel as a result of reading our welcome pack – and that this is a good outcome.

❒ When customers arrive we ask for the completed initial paperwork, plus a specific request to complete the menu.

Congratulations on completing *The Customer Journey 100*! Revisit the programme until you get 100 ticks. Remember, every professional's experience will be different. Be kind to yourself and work at your own pace. There is no one right way to reach 100! Good luck.

Index